Adverse Drug Reactions

A Practical Guide to Diagnosis and Management

Adverse Drug Reactions

A Practical Guide to Diagnosis and Management

Edited by
Christian Bénichou
International Department of Drug Safety,
Roussel Uclaf, Paris, France

translated by éditions pradel

JOHN WILEY & SONS
Chichester · New York · Brisbane · Toronto · Singapore

Copyright © 1994 by John Wiley & Sons Ltd,
Baffins Lane, Chichester,
West Sussex PO19 1UD, England
Telephone: National Chichester (01243) 779777
International +44 1243 779777

Reprinted July 1995, November 1995, August 1996

First published by éditions pradel, France 1992

Other Wiley Editorial Offices

John Wiley & Sons, Inc., 605 Third Avenue,
New York, NY 10158-0012, USA

Jacaranda Wiley Ltd, 33 Park Road, Milton,
Queensland 4064, Australia

John Wiley & Sons (Canada) Ltd, 22 Worcester Road,
Rexdale, Ontario M9W 1L1, Canada

John Wiley & Sons (SEA) Pte Ltd, 37 Jalan Pemimpin #05-04,
Block B, Union Industrial Building, Singapore 2057

Library of Congress Cataloging-in-Publication Data

Guide pratique de pharmacovigilance. English.
    Adverse drug reactions: a practical guide to diagnosis and
    management/edited by Christian Bénichou: translated by Éditions Pradel.
      p.   cm.
    Includes bibliographical references and index.
    ISBN 0 471 94211 1.
    1. Drugs—Side effects—Reporting.   I. Bénichou, Christian.   II. Title.
    [DNLM: 1. Drugs—adverse effects.   2. Drug Hypersensitivity—
diagnosis.   3. Drug Hypersensitivity—therapy.   4. Adverse Drug
Reaction Reporting Systems.   QV 38 G9457 1994a]
RM302.5.G8413   1994
615'.704—dc20
DNLM/DLC
for Library of Congress   94-6102
                                                                    CIP

British Library Cataloguing in Publication Data

A catalogue record for this book is available from the British Library

ISBN 0 471 94211 1

Typeset by Dobbie Typesetting
Printed and bound in Great Britain by
Biddles Ltd, Guildford and King's Lynn

Authors

Christian BÉNICHOU, MD
Director, International Drug Monitoring Department, Roussel Uclaf, Paris

Pierre BOUCHE, MD
Consultant in Neurology, Pitié Salpêtrière Hospital, Paris

Jacques CARON, MD
Consultant in Cardiology, University Hospital Center, Lille

Catherine CHAPELON, MD
Consultant in Cardiology, Pitié Salpêtrière Hospital, Paris

Gaby DANAN, MD
International Drug Monitoring Department, Roussel Uclaf, Paris.
Consultant in Hepatology, Beaujon Hospital, Clichy

Didier DEFFOND, MD
Consultant in Neurology, Regional Hospital Center, Clermont-Ferrand

Gérard DORDAIN, MD
Professor, Department of Neurology, Regional Hospital Center, Clermont-Ferrand

Ralph EDWARDS, MD
Professor, Medical Director, WHO Collaborating Center for International Drug Monitoring, Uppsala

Antoine FLAHAULT, MD, PhD
Consultant in Epidemiology, International Drug Monitoring Department, Roussel Uclaf, Paris

Michel FOURNIER, MD
Professor, Department of Pneumology, Beaujon Hospital, Clichy

Alex PARIENTE, MD
Consultant in Hepatology and Gastro-Enterology, Regional Hospital Center, Pau

Eugène ROTHSCHILD, MD
International Drug Monitoring Department, Roussel Uclaf, Paris.
Consultant in Nephrology, Necker Hospital, Paris

Jean-Claude ROUJEAU, MD
Professor, Department of Dermatology, Henri Mondor Hospital, Créteil

Philippe SOLAL-CELIGNY, MD
Victor Hugo Oncoradiotherapy and Hematology Center, Le Mans. Department of Hematology, Saint-Louis Hospital, Paris

Georges TCHOBROUTSKY, MD
Professor, Department of Diabetology, Hôtel Dieu Hospital, Paris

Didier VERNAY, MD
Consultant in Neurology, Regional Hospital Center, Clermont-Ferrand

Ernst WEIDMANN, MD
Director, Corporate Drug Safety Department, Hoechst AG, Frankfurt

The authors gratefully acknowledge the painstaking and skillful assistance of Christine André and Mireille Vanthuyne for the preparation and make-up of this edition.

They wish to thank particularly Dr Myles Stephens for reviewing the English edition and for his relevant suggestions based on his wide and well known experience in drug safety.

Contents

Foreword

Could it be drug-related?

This is not a question that arises when explaining improvement in a patient who is receiving drugs. Recent decades have brought such profound changes in the course and prognosis of diseases that were sometimes or always fatal that the benefits of modern therapies are obvious, the most easily quantifiable aspect of these being the increased life expectancy that the patient can now expect.

Nowadays, the focus tends to be more on the hazards of drugs rather than on their benefits. No mention is made of medicines in connection with their curative effects, but their failures or adverse reactions make the headlines. Both aspects, efficacy and safety, are of equal importance. They should never be separated when evaluating the merits of a drug or a class of therapeutic agents, that is to say, when undertaking a collective risk–benefit assessment that, theoretically, is a summation of individual risk–benefit analyses. However on an individual level, the assessment may reach just the opposite conclusion: a generally well-tolerated broad-spectrum antibiotic may present nothing but disadvantages for the patient infected by a bacterium resistant to that antibiotic. Therefore, it is not enough to consider only the situation in the majority of cases; for minorities and individuals, the all-or-none law applies as regards safety as well as efficacy.

No doubt, this accounts for the different approaches of manufacturers or regulatory agencies, on one side, and prescribers and patients on the other. A patient will be hard put to understand why he was prescribed a drug that produced a reaction more severe than the illness for which he was treated. Another patient will not accept the fact that he is being denied a drug that had brought him relief for years without causing any apparent problem whatsoever. Some prescribers believe that they have sufficient experience with medications whose negative aspects they have never encountered. Others are surprised by the frequency or severity of adverse reactions that by chance have affected a small number of their own patients. Prescribers form the foundation upon which the entire edifice rests: practically all major but uncommon adverse reactions have been discovered through spontaneous reporting by practising physicians. Without them, pharmacovigilance would be impossible, and disasters such as the one caused by thalidomide would be repeated. In return, they must be kept informed not only of decisions concerning drugs but also of the reasons that led up to those decisions, if we want them to be understood and applied efficiently. A drug is more dangerous when its use in a patient is prolonged unduly because its toxicity has not been recognized. No signal can be neglected. Validated information must be distributed rapidly to all parties concerned whose roles in this regard are complementary.

Christian Bénichou

Introduction

Pharmacovigilance: a crucial activity

Clinical trials do not involve large enough series of patients and these patients are not treated for a sufficiently long period to guarantee the detection of all the adverse effects of the study medication: the adverse effects may be rare or delayed or result from interactions with other drugs, or may only put at risk a subgroup of patients. It is therefore essential to monitor a drug after marketing. Pharmacovigilance, a term originally applied only to the unexpected effects of marketed drugs, has an increasingly important place in the establishment of the risk–benefit assessment of a drug.

Spontaneous reporting, "mandatory" in France since 1984, is an irreplaceable source of information in pharmacovigilance: rare and/or delayed severe adverse reactions would have gone unnoticed were it not for the discernment and critical thinking of clinicians who were surprised by the appearance of an adverse event, considered its possible relationship to a drug, collected the evidence in support of such a relationship, and decided to transmit the information to the regulatory agencies or manufacturers who could make use of the data. Intensive studies or cohorts are very costly and can never include enough patients to discover unfailingly those adverse reactions whose incidence is less than 1 per 5000 or 10 000 patients. Therefore, the solution to this public health problem is dependent in large measure on the alertness and goodwill of medical practitioners.

The training or awareness of the practising physician is not always adequate for this task. Not all prescribers could possibly be turned into experts in the evaluation of the causal relationship between a drug and an adverse clinical event. Actually, the assessment of the role of a drug is only one aspect of the classic medical diagnostic process, which includes a differential diagnosis and an etiologic diagnosis. The latter, as far as drugs are concerned, is based on evidence for or against a temporal relationship—the timing of the event—and on ruling out the other principal non-drug-related causes of the event observed.

Chronological criteria are of the utmost importance in pharmacovigilance. The most obvious and least questionable link between a drug and an event is the timing between first administration of the drug and onset of the event: an event that began prior to the start of a treatment cannot be due to that treatment. On the contrary, when certain events appear within minutes or hours of the administration of an agent, there is a fair likelihood that they were caused by that agent; when the interval is measured in days or weeks, the probability of a causal relationship will depend on the event. The course of the event over time, according to whether the administration of the drug is continued or discontinued, will provide meaningful data: a reaction that disappears while the treatment is still ongoing has little chance of being drug-related; a reaction that recurs in exactly the same way, without reintroduction of the drug, several days or weeks following its discontinuation is unlikely to have been caused by that drug. A reaction that reappears after a drug is reintroduced has a very strong likelihood of being related to it. These commonsense considerations are applied daily in the practice of pharmacovigilance. For a valid analysis to be performed, very precise temporal data must be supplied, in terms of the date, and even the hour, on which the administration of a drug started and ended, or of the time sequence between the start and the end of a treatment and the occurrence of an adverse clinical event.

The investigation of non-drug-related causes is of greater or lesser importance according to the share attributable to medicines in the etiology of the adverse experience; when medicines play only a small part, the search for other causes is of fundamental importance. But at this point this share has to be well-defined for each type of event. This will have to be done, and a list will have to be made of the pertinent investigations for evaluating the non-drug-drelated causes.

In this book, we have collected a number of facts pertaining to most of the important adverse drug reactions. This has been made possible through the contributions of consultants in different medical fields, including colleagues who work with us regularly, and also outside consultants. With the cooperation of some of these contributors, consensus meetings were able to be organized on the definitions and causality assessment criteria in pharmacovigilance, of which more will be said further on.

This book is intended for medical practitioners, but it may also be helpful to professionals who specialize in pharmacovigilance: the areas included in this field of activity are as varied as those of medicine, and no one could claim to be an expert in all areas Although we did not consider every type of adverse reaction, most of the reactions that are likely to affect the profile of use of a drug have been included.

Considerable space has been devoted in these pages to guidelines for appropriate action in the event of meeting in practice an abnormal clinical or laboratory finding that may possibly be drug-related: how to establish a positive diagnosis based on the definition and criteria of severity of the abnormality; how to direct the etiological investigations bearing in mind the relative frequency of a drug-related cause for the clinical event, the tests for assessing the nondrug causes and the diagnostic criteria for the role of drugs; whether to stop the drug or to continue its administration, or whether urgent hospitalization in a specialized department is necessary. Therapeutic trials are discussed in a special chapter. The circumstances may vary: the subjects are often already in hospital and are being closely monitored.

The advice given in this book reflects the thinking of drug toxicity specialists in different fields. These recommendations cannot be considered as official, and each prescriber or investigator can and must discontinue the administration of a drug if he deems it best to do so.

Among the editorial problems that were encountered, three particular issues should be mentioned:

- The length of the texts: while the purpose was not to compile an encyclopedic review, it was also necessary to avoid limiting the discussions to generalities so broad that they would lose any practical value.

- The mention of product names involves delicate choices: fairly often, only therapeutic classes or chemical families are cited. The different chapters were assigned to authors under their own responsibility; the texts reflect their opinion, as in any scientific publication, but are generally in keeping with published compilations of approved product information.

- Guidelines: although it would not be possible to deal with every situation, this work would lose much of its value if it contained no practical advice for the medical practitioner. We chose to offer guidelines pertinent to the largest number of cases, especially in emergency situations.

- To allow a fast reading, many texts have been presented in two columns, the left one giving the essential information, the right one comments on complementary explanations.

Consensus meetings on adverse drug reactions:
The need for standardization and harmonization

The sources of information in pharmacovigilance are diverse: spontaneous reports, studies and publications in scientific journals. The numerous countries of origin do not always share the same concepts of disease classification and definition. The information supplied by the reporter may be collected at the local level and then transmitted to the company headquarters, where it will be evaluated and classified according to the constraints of a thesaurus, and sent on subsequently to one or more regulatory agencies at a national level, each of which has its own methods of data management.

In order to retrieve and group together medically related or similar clinical entities, terminologies have been proposed for adverse reactions, the most widely distributed being the one published by the World Health Organization (WHO ART). These are lists of terms without definitions. If we compare the definitions of these terms in different medical dictionaries, we find that reference works do not always agree with each other, that they do not always take age-related variations into account, and that, to be used, they often require complete information, rarely available in pharmacovigilance. Therefore, it is necessary to have definitions that are accepted by the different parties involved and can be used in conjunction with a certain level of documentation. The objective is to ensure that no information likely to add to our knowledge of a drug will be omitted, and that imprecise or meaningless data can be identified as such.

Moreover, many causality assessment methods have been proposed to evaluate the role of a drug in the development of an adverse drug reaction. Criteria to assess the causal relationship are common to most methods: chronological relationship between the administration of the drug and the occurrence of the event, screening for non-drug-related causes, confirmation of the reaction in *in vivo* or *in vitro* tests, and previous information on similar events attributed to the suspect drug or to its therapeutic class. No single method has been universally adopted. The qualities usually required for a causality assessment method are reproducibility and validity. Reproducibility ensures an identical result, regardless of the method's user, and when he/she uses it. Validity means the ability of the method to distinguish between cases where the drug is responsible and cases where it is not. The low reproducibility of these methods, the principal criticism leveled at them, can be explained by the fact that the limits of the timing criteria or the principal alternative causes to be considered are left to the judgment of each evaluator.

Thus, there seems to be a need to agree upon and to standardize the definitions and evaluation criteria for adverse reactions. Roussel Uclaf has organized national, and subsequently international, consensus meetings whose purposes were to arrive at definitions of adverse reactions tailored to the quality of information usually available in pharmacovigilance, and to propose a choice of precise terms adapted to each of the reactions for the criteria common to the different methods. Three fields of endeavor involved in pharmacovigilance were represented at the meetings: hospital and university experts; representatives from the French pharmacovigilance system; and members of the Roussel Uclaf Pharmacovigilance Department. One or more meetings with French experts were held to deal with each of the following subjects: liver impairment, granulocytopenia or thrombocytopenia, hemolytic anemia, renal failure, interstitial lung disorders, vascular purpura and photosensitivity.

The process of the consensus meetings may be illustrated by the example of drug-induced liver disorders: two meetings were organized in 1985 and 1986 with nine French participants. They had to answer four basic questions:

a) Is the liver involved? (When histological data are lacking, diagnosis depends on the result of biochemical tests.)

b) How should liver test abnormalities be classified?

c) Which chronological and clinical criteria suggest a drug-induced reaction?

d) What are the nondrug related causes and how should they be ruled out?

Later, at the request of the Council for International Organizations of Medical Sciences (CIOMS), international meetings were organized to deal with drug-induced hepatic reactions and blood cytopenias. The first part of each meeting was devoted, again, to the definitions and classification of the different abnormal clinical or laboratory findings, and the second part to the criteria for evaluating the role of the drug. For each of the criteria, the study group was asked to consider a list of qualifying terms characterizing the degree of probability that the drug could have induced the adverse event. To adapt the weight of each criterion to each reaction, not all these categories of terms necessarily had to be used, but only the ones that appeared to correspond most closely to the experience of the experts. In addition, all possible time sequences, with precise limits, had to be covered by the categories of terms selected.

Regarding liver disorders, the participants included eight experts in hepatology from six countries: JP Benhamou (France), L Bircher (Germany), G Danan (France), WC Maddrey (USA), J Neuberger (UK), F Orlandi (Italy), N Tygstrup (Denmark) and HJ Zimmerman (USA). A few weeks before the meeting, all participants received the conclusions of the French meeting and a list of 13 questions. As the participants had been given several weeks to prepare the answers to the questions, they understood the nature of the compromise that this type of situation imposes.

Concerning the chronological criteria, the experts had to consider the time interval between the beginning *or* the end of administration of the drug and the occurrence of the event; and, regarding the course of the event, to distinguish the consequences of discontinuation *or* continuation of the drug. The proposed adjectives were:

Time to onset: 'highly suggestive', 'suggestive', 'compatible', 'inconclusive', 'incompatible' (meaning that the causal relationship could definitively be ruled out)

Course of the reaction: 'highly suggestive', 'suggestive', 'compatible', 'against the role of the drug' (but this situation cannot rule out a role for the drug) or 'inconclusive'

Regarding other criteria, the experts were also asked to list the following:

• factors known to increase the risk of occurrence of the event

- main non drug-related causes and the relevant tests to be performed
- laboratory tests or drug plasma concentrations enabling confirmation of the causal role of a drug
- conditions required to assess the response to reintroduction of a suspect drug that was thought to have induced the same reaction after a previous administration

The meeting on blood cytopenias involved eight experts in hematology from five countries: E Baumelou (France), B Camitta (USA), L Degos (France), EC Gordon Smith (UK), H Heimpel (Germany), P Solal Céligny (France), PC Vincent (Australia) and N Young (USA).

The conclusions arrived at during the consensus meetings are presented in this book in the form of tables at the end of each chapter. In addition, a new method for causality assessment of drugs, based on the conclusions of the meetings, and its application to drug-induced acute liver disorders, is presented in Chapter 22.

References

Bénichou C, Danan G. Lack of definitions of adverse drug reactions. Drugs Inform J 1989; 23: 71–4.

Bénichou C, Solal Céligny P. Standardization of definitions and criteria for causality assessment of adverse drug reactions. Drug-induced blood cytopenias. Report of an International Consensus Meeting. Nouv Rev Fr Hematol 1991; 33: 257–62.

Danan G. Consensus meeting on causality assessment of drug-induced liver injury. J Hepatol 1988; 7: 132–6.

Fournier M, Camus P, Bénichou C, et al. Pneumopathies interstitielles. Critères d'imputation à un médicament. Résultats de réunions de consensus. Press Med 1989; 18: 1333–6.

Guillaume JC, Roujeau JC, Chevrant-Breton J, et al. Comment imputer un accident cutané à un médicament. Application aux purpuras vasculaires. Ann Dermatol Venereol 1987; 114: 721–4.

Habibi B, Solal Céligny P, Bénichou C, et al. Anémies hémolytiques d'origine médicamenteuse. Résultats de réunions de consensus. Thérapie 1988; 43: 117–20.

International Consensus Meeting. Criteria of drug-induced liver disorders. J Hepatol 1990; 11: 272–6.

Roujeau JC, Béani JC, Dubertret L, et al. Photosensibilité cutanée médicamenteuse. Résultats d'une réunion de consensus. Thérapie 1989; 44: 223–7.

Solal Céligny P, Bénichou C, Boivin P, et al. Critères d'imputation d'une cytopénie granuleuse ou plaquettaire à un médicament. Résultats de réunions de consensus. Nouv Rev Fr Hematol 1987; 29: 265–70.

Vigeral P, Baumelou A, Bénichou C, et al. Les insuffisances rénales d'origine médicamenteuse. Résultats de réunions de consensus. Nephrologie 1989; 10: 157–61.

PART I

Diagnosis and Management of Adverse Drug Reactions

1 Liver test abnormalities

Gaby Danan

If liver damage is suspected, the first tests to order are serum assays of the transaminases SGPT (ALT) and SGOT (AST), alkaline phosphatase, and total and conjugated (direct) bilirubin.

Transaminases

Any transaminase elevation above the upper limit of normal for the laboratory **should be considered**.

Since the reference values (normal values) vary with the laboratory that performed the assay, it is desirable that the serum transaminase level should be expressed as a multiple of N (the upper limit of normal).

Is it of hepatic origin?

Yes, if the ALT level is elevated.

In practice, an elevation in ALT is considered specific for liver damage.

Not always if the level of AST alone is elevated.

Elevated AST may be due to muscle damage; this is why it is necessary to make sure that CPK activity is normal. However, the relation of elevated AST activity to liver involvement can be confirmed if it is associated with an elevation in alkaline phosphatase activity or conjugated bilirubin.

Alkaline phosphatase

Any rise in alkaline phosphatase above the upper limit of normal for the laboratory **should be considered**.

Since the reference values (normal values) vary with the laboratory that performed the assay, it is desirable

Adverse Drug Reactions. A Practical Guide to Diagnosis and Management. Edited by C. Bénichou.
©1994 John Wiley & Sons Ltd.

that the serum alkaline phosphatase activity should be expressed as a multiple of N (the upper limit of normal).

Is it of hepatic origin?

Yes, if there is a concomitant elevation in gamma glutamyl transpeptidase (GGT), in ALT, or in conjugated bilirubin.

The associated 5'-nucleotidase elevation, specific to cholestasis, is delayed and less sensitive.

Not always, because their **isolated** elevation is seen in other diseases.

For example, Paget's disease, bone metastases.

Definitions

Can any liver damage be called hepatitis?

Strictly speaking, hepatitis is a histologic lesion of the liver characterized by an infiltration of mononuclear cells that may or may not be associated with hepatocellular changes. Therefore, this term should be reserved for cases in which a histologic evaluation has been performed, while the term "liver injury" should be used in other cases.

The term "hepatitis" is misused or loosely used to refer to any liver damage, whether or not histologic lesions of the liver are present.

*It is not necessary to perform a liver biopsy to be certain of a hepatic reaction (see transaminases, alkaline phosphatase). A biopsy becomes **necessary** when the therapeutic decision depends on the nature of the lesion.*

The occurrence of jaundice and/or a transaminase elevation above 2 N and/or an alkaline phosphatase elevation above 1.5 N necessitates:

- **withdrawal** of all medications not vital to life*
- **surveillance** of the abnormalities at least once a week
- **search** for some other cause, primarily:
  - a viral infection or acute hypotension, in the case of hepatocellular injury
  - biliary tract obstruction, in the case of cholestatic injury

---

* If you are in doubt concerning the hepatotoxicity of a drug considered essential, consult a specialist in hepatology or pharmacovigilance.

What type of liver injury?

Regardless of what the exact nature of the histologic lesions of the liver turns out to be, the injury should be classified as **hepatocellular, cholestatic** or **mixed**, because the prognosis depends upon it.

The classification is based on the ratio:

$$R = \frac{\text{ALT value}}{\text{alkaline phosphatase value}}$$

Ratio R should be calculated as soon as the abnormalities are observed because it may vary over time, as some hepatocellular injuries are complicated by cholestasis. The enzymes should all be assayed at the same time.

The values for each of the enzymes are expressed in N (upper limit of normal) and values below the upper limit of normal are considered equal to N.

hepatocellular injury: isolated elevation of transaminases of hepatic origin or $R \geqslant 5$.

Hepatocellular injury generally reflects liver necrosis; in the case of jaundice, it is life-threatening.

cholestatic injury: isolated elevation of alkaline phosphatase of hepatic origin or $R \leqslant 2$.

Cholestatic injury—cessation or reduction of bile secretion—is potentially less serious in the short term, even if jaundice is present. However, it may take several weeks or months to resolve.

mixed (combined) damage: concomitant elevation of transaminases and alkaline phosphatase and $2 < R < 5$.

The prognosis in mixed injury is similar to that of cholestatic injury.

Acute or chronic hepatic injury?

Liver injury is **acute** when the liver function test abnormalities last less than three months; it is **chronic** when they last more than three months.

Signs of severity

In increasing order of severity:
- jaundice, in the case of hepatocellular injury

The presence of one of these signs calls for immediate hospitalization in a specialized department.

- prothrombin time (PT) < 50%
  together with factor V (proaccelerin)
  < 50%
- hepatic encephalopathy, the first
  stage of which is characterized by
  asterixis (a flapping tremor).

Evidence implicating a drug

- The adverse event is **very probably** drug-related if reintroduction of the drug is again followed by the same reaction. Rechallenge (intentional reintroduction) is ethically unacceptable because of its potentially life-threatening consequences, and the re-administration of the drug has usually been unintentional.
- The adverse event is **probably** drug-related if the other principal causes were able to be ruled out (see below).
- In the other cases, the role of the drug is only **possible** or **unlikely**.
- However, there are only two circumstances in which a relationship with the drug can be **excluded**:
  - If the timing is incompatible, i.e. in the following situations:
    - when drug administration follows the onset of liver damage.
    - when the liver abnormalities are discovered more than two weeks after the drug is withdrawn,* in the case of hepatocellular damage, or one month with cholestatic damage.
    - If a non drug-related cause is proved.

Etiology

Overall, in acute liver damage, it is estimated that the event is drug-related in about 10% of cases. After the age of 50, the proportion is approximately 50%.

Individual susceptibility or the illness being treated may be responsible for abnormal liver test findings

Chronic alcoholism

Elevated transaminase levels are generally due to fatty liver or acute alcoholic hepatitis, which may or may not be associated with cirrhosis.

Fatty liver is often detectable by ultrasound examination. Acute alcoholic hepatitis can be confirmed only by histologic examination of liver biopsy.

---

*Except if drug clearance is very slow.

Although alcoholism is common, liver test abnormalities should not be attributed to it automatically, and a careful search should be made for some other cause—particularly relating to a drug—which may necessitate asking the opinion of a specialist.

Elevated transaminase levels with a AST/ALT ratio greater than 2 is suggestive of alcoholic liver damage.

Bacterial infection

Bacterial infection sometimes produces an elevation of alkaline phosphatase or serum bilirubin. Transaminase levels are more rarely elevated and only exceptionally exceed 5 N.

These abnormalities are more frequent and of greater magnitude (jaundice) in cases of severe infection (septicemia) or when the causative organism is a gram-negative bacillus or pneumococcus.

Right-sided heart failure

Right-sided (or biventricular) heart failure may produce congestion of the liver with ensuing moderate elevations of alkaline phosphatase and/or transaminases and/or of bilirubin unconjugated in most instances.

Hepatomegaly and hepatojugular reflux are generally present. These abnormalities regress with the treatment of heart failure.

Left-sided heart-failure or fall in blood pressure

A severe blood pressure drop, or left-sided (or biventricular) heart failure, when complicated by an acute event (arrhythmia or infarction) that reduces the cardiac output, may result in stagnant **hypoxia of the liver** reflected by a precipitous rise in serum transaminase levels followed by a rapid return to normal. When hyperbilirubinemia occurs, it is delayed by 48–72 hours.

The diagnosis is based on:

- *a known drop in blood pressure (or its consequences), even if temporary, in the 24–48 hour period preceding the abnormalities;*
- *very rapid transaminase changes;*
- *elevated blood urea nitrogen and/or plasma creatinine levels;*
- *other signs of tissue anoxia (particularly, increased CPK).*

Examination shows no liver enlargement or hepatojugular reflux.

This picture resembles acute drug-induced hepatocellular damage in every respect. This diagnosis must be considered routinely in this setting.

These abnormalities are greater as the anoxia is more prolonged. The outcome may be fatal, especially in elderly patients.

Other causes of liver damage

What are the principal tests to be ordered?

In hepatocellular injury

- Tests for serum markers of a recent viral infection:

  — with hepatitis A virus: anti-HAV IgM

  The presence of anti-HAV IgG would indicate an old infection.

  — with hepatitis B virus: anti-HBc IgM

  This is the only specific marker for a recent infection with hepatitis B virus.

  — with CMV: anti-CMV IgM; with EBV: Paul-Bunnell test (or, better, anti-VCA IgM).

  Only if the setting is indicative of it: e.g. mononucleosis.

  — with hepatitis C virus: antibody to HCV, but its **late** appearance requires a search for circumstantial evidence of infection with hepatitis C virus (former non-A, non-B transmitted parenterally) or hepatitis E virus (former non-A, non-B transmitted enterally).

  Within the past six months:

  - *transfusion of blood or of blood products (generally within 8 weeks)*
  - *intravenous drug abuse*
  - *localized epidemic context*
  - *recent travel, particularly to Africa, Asia, India.*

  This marker:

  — is present only in 70% of cases due to hepatitis C virus;

  — is absent during the acute phase: it appears only after the second or even the fourth month, so the tests have to be repeated.

- Hepatobiliary ultrasound examination

  Especially to detect an acute temporary biliary obstruction by a stone.

- Tests for antinuclear, anti-DNA and anti-smooth muscle autoantibodies

  In support of autoimmune chronic active hepatitis, a disease with a female preponderance; liver biopsy is necessary.

In cholestatic injury

- Hepatobiliary ultrasound examination

  To detect biliary obstruction (even partial). In case of doubt, direct opacification of the biliary tract must be performed.

- Test for serum markers of virus infection (see above)

- Test for antimitochondrial and also for antinuclear, anti-DNA and anti-smooth muscle antibodies.

A high titer of antimitochondrial antibodies is indicative of primary biliary cirrhosis.

Immunologic tests in the presence of drug, such as the *in vitro* lymphoblast transformation test, the test of inhibition of leukocyte migration or the human basophil degranulation test, are **not at all helpful** for diagnosing drug-induced origin.

Conclusion

If the search for a non drug-related origin is negative:

- a drug-induced cause is probable, but the hepatotoxic agent may be difficult to identify;
- the suspect drugs must never again be administered, and the patient should be informed of this.

References

Dhumeaux D. Hépatite non-A, non-B, type C. Gastroenterol Clin Biol 1990; 14: T26–9.

International Consensus Meeting. Criteria of drug-induced liver disorders. J Hepatol 1990; 11: 272–6.

Pessayre D, Larrey D, Benhamou JP. Hépatites médicamenteuses. Semaine des Hôpitaux de Paris 1985; 61: 2049–71.

DESIGNATIONS OF DRUG-INDUCED LIVER DISORDERS ON BASIS OF ABNORMALITIES SHOWN BY LIVER TESTS

TERMS REQUIRING HISTOLOGICAL DATA

Hepatitis
Hepatic necrosis
Chronic liver disease
Cirrhosis

IN THE ABSENCE OF HISTOLOGICAL DATA

→**Abnormalities of liver tests**

Any increase between N and 2N in
- ALT
- or AST
- or AP
- or TB

→**Liver injury**

- Increase over 2N in ALT or CB
- or combined increase in AST, AP and TB, providing one of them is above 2N

TYPE OF LIVER INJURY

- **Hepatocellular:** increase over 2N in ALT alone, **or** $R \geqslant 5$
- **Cholestatic:** increase over 2N in AP, **or** $R \leqslant 2$
- **Mixed:** increase of both ALT over 2N and AP, and $2 < R < 5$
- **Acute:** Elevation of liver tests lasting less than three months
- **Chronic:** Elevation of liver tests lasting more than three months
- **Fulminant:** Rapid (days to weeks) development of hepatic encephalopathy and severe coagulation disorders
- **Severe:** Liver injury complicated by, in order of increasing severity: jaundice, prothrombin < 50%, hepatic encephalopathy

SYMBOLS

ALT* = Alanine aminotransferase
AST** = Aspartate aminotransferase
N = Upper limit of the normal range

AP = Alkaline phosphatase
CB = Conjugated bilirubin
TB = Total bilirubin

$$(\text{ratio}) \ R = \frac{\text{Serum activity of ALT}}{\text{Serum activity of AP}}$$

(Each activity is expressed as a multiple of N. Both should be measured together at the time of recognition of liver injury.)

*(formerly SGPT)
**(formerly SGOT)

ACUTE HEPATOCELLULAR LIVER DAMAGE
CHRONOLOGICAL CRITERIA

		Very suggestive	Suggestive	Compatible		Inconclusive	Incompatible	
Time to onset of the reaction	Initial treatment		*From start of drug administration* 5–90 days	*From start of drug administration* <5 days or >90 days	*From end of drug administration** ≤15 days		*With regard to start of drug administration* Drug taken after the onset of the reaction	*From end of drug administration* >15 days except for slowly metabolized drugs
	Subsequent treatment with or without previous history of acute liver injury in relation to the same drug		*From start of drug administration* 1–15 days	*From start of drug administration* >15 days				

*Or from the time at which the drug is supposed to have been cleared from the body.

		Very suggestive	Suggestive	Compatible	Inconclusive	Not suggestive
Course of the reaction	Without stopping the drug				All situations	
	After stopping the drug	Decrease of ALT* ≥50% of the excess over N† within 8 days and no additional elevation of ALT within 30 days	Decrease of ALT≥50% of the excess over N within 30 days		No information on the course of liver tests	Other variations of ALT

*ALT (or SGPT) = alanine aminotransferase; †N = upper limit of normal range.

ACUTE CHOLESTATIC OR MIXED LIVER DAMAGE
CHRONOLOGICAL CRITERIA

		Very suggestive	Suggestive	Compatible	Inconclusive	Incompatible
Time to onset of the reaction	Initial treatment		*From start of drug administration* 5–90 days	*From start of drug administration* <5 days or >90 days	*From end of drug administration* ≤30 days	*From end of drug administration* >30 days
	Subsequent treatment with or without previous history of acute liver injury in relation to the same drug		*From start of drug administration* 1–90 days	*From start of drug administration* >90 days		*With regard to start of drug administration* Drug taken after the onset of the reaction

		Very suggestive	Suggestive	Compatible	Inconclusive	Not suggestive
Course of the reaction	Without stopping the drug				All situations	
	After stopping the drug		Decrease of AP* or TB† ≥50% of the excess over N‡ within 6 months	Decrease of AP or TB <50% of the excess over N within 6 months	AP or TB levels: stable or increased or no information on the course of liver tests	

*AP = alkaline phosphatase; †TB = total bilirubin; ‡N = upper limit of normal range.

2 Abnormal hematologic values

Philippe Solal-Céligny

Neutropenia and agranulocytosis

This chapter does not cover neutropenia and agranulocytosis related to cytotoxic agents used for cancer or antiviral chemotherapy, which are predictable and generally pose no diagnostic problem.

Definitions

Neutropenia: polymorphonuclear neutrophil (PMN) count below 1500/μL (1.5 × 10⁹/L).

Epidemiological surveys in Africa have demonstrated that normal black subjects may have a PMN count of less than 1500/μL.

Severe neutropenia: PMN count lower than 500/μL (0.5 × 10⁹/L).

The term **agranulocytosis** is reserved for a situation in which the abrupt onset of severe neutropenia is associated with clinical signs, including fever, severe asthenia and buccopharyngeal and/or perineal ulcers.

leukopenia (white blood cell count below 3000/μL) should be used only if a differential count has not been done.

Management

Neutropenia without signs of severity or risk factors

- Discontinue drugs not essential for life.
- Conduct a careful search for an incipient infection.

Signs of severity:

- *fever*
- *symptoms and/or signs of infection.*

Risk factors for infection include:

- *recent surgical operations*
- *urinary or biliary obstruction*

Adverse Drug Reactions. A Practical Guide to Diagnosis and Management. Edited by C. Bénichou.
©1994 John Wiley & Sons Ltd.

- Perform a complete blood count 48 hours later.
- Obtain the advice of a specialist if the disease persists or if the neutrophil count falls further subsequently.

- *chronic obstructive pulmonary disease*
- *HIV infection*
- *immunosuppressive therapy*

Agranulocytosis or neutropenia with signs of severity or risk factors

- Discontinue drugs not essential for life.
- Except in special circumstances, hospitalization is necessary to monitor the patient closely and so that a bone marrow examination can be performed in order to:
  - study the marrow cellularity and more particularly that of the granulocytic series
  - search for infiltrative tumor cells.
- If **fever** is present:
  - perform blood cultures
  - take local specimens (urine, throat, skin lesions, etc.)
  - look for a respiratory infection
  - **immediately** institute **intravenous** broad-spectrum antibiotic therapy with several **bactericidal** agents.

Evidence implicating a drug

Isolated neutropenia = neutropenia without involvement of the other blood cells (red blood cells, platelets).

In the presence of isolated neutropenia, a drug-related origin should be considered immediately. However, the diagnosis can be established only by the outcome and by ruling out nondrug causes.

Search for nondrug causes

- Viral infections

  - *human immunodeficiency virus*
  - *Epstein–Barr virus*
  - *cytomegalovirus, rubella, varicella*

- Bacterial infections

  - *typhoid fever*
  - *brucellosis*

- Systemic diseases

  - *systemic lupus erythematosus*
  - *collagen diseases*
  - *rheumatoid arthritis*

- Blood disorders

  - *hairy-cell leukemia*
  - *suppressor T-cell leukemia*
  - *myelodysplastic syndrome (refractory anemia)*

- Autoimmune neutropenia
- Toxic agents

- *benzene derivatives*
- *ionizing radiations*

A drug-related etiology is more probable when:

- The neutropenia is **recent**

Previous CBCs of great importance

- The **bone marrow examination** shows:
  - hypocellular or regenerating granulocytic series
  - normal morphology of the different precursors
  - absence of abnormal infiltration by hematopoietic or extrahematopoietic cells.

Regenerating marrow = predominance of young forms (promyelocytes, myelocytes) over late forms (metamyelocytes, polymorphonuclears) of neutrophil precursors

- The drug is known to have **caused** neutropenia

Refer to latest information supplied by manufacturer in the PDR or local drug dictionary

- The neutropenia is **reversible** on discontinuation of the drug.

Drug-induced neutropenia nearly always resolves on withdrawal of the offending drug:
- *usually within 6 weeks, sometimes more slowly*
- *generally, recovery is complete*
- *without recurrence, unless the offending agent is reintroduced.*

- *In vitro* **tests** indicative of "**immunoallergic**" **neutropenia** are positive. There are two principal types of tests:
  - demonstration in the patient's serum of antibodies that bind to autologous polymorphonuclear cells only in the presence of the drug;
  - inhibition of the growth of bone marrow granulocytic progenitors (CFU_{GM}: colony forming unit granulocyte-macrophage) by the combination of the serum and the drug.

Blood collection and preservation procedure: collect a serum specimen 3–5 days after discontinuing the drug (the sample may be frozen)

- **Nonspecific tests** for anti-drug immunity are of no value in the study of drug-induced neutropenia.

For example:
- *lymphocyte transformation test*
- *test of inhibition of leukocyte migration*
- *basophil degranulation test*

The absence of one or more of these criteria does not rule out a drug-related origin.

The great majority of severe, acute, isolated, reversible neutropenias are drug-induced.

Such cases have been described with certain drugs in most therapeutic classes.

Some classes are involved more frequently:
- pyrazolone derivatives
- antidepressants
- antithyroid drugs
- penicillamine
- beta-lactam antibiotics
- sulfonamides
- nonsteroidal antiinflammatory drugs

References

Bénichou C, Solal-Céligny P. Standardization of definitions and criteria for causality assessment of adverse drug reactions. Drug-induced blood cytopenias. Report of an International Consensus Meeting. Nouv Rev Fh Hematol 1991; 33: 257–62.

Heimpel H. Drug-induced agranulocytosis. Adverse drug experience review. Medical Toxicology 1988; 3: 449-62.

Pisciotta AV. Drug induced agranulocytosis. Peripheral destruction of polymorphonuclear leukocytes and their marrow precursors. Blood Reviews 1990; 4: 226–37.

The International Agranulocytosis and Aplastic Anemia Study. Anti-infective drug use in relation to the risk of agranulocytosis and aplastic anemia. Arch Intern Med 1989; 149: 1036–40.

Thrombocytopenia*

Definition

Platelet count below 100 000/μL

When the count ranges from 100 000 to 150 000/μL, there is no risk of bleeding provided platelet function is normal, but blood counts must be performed on the subsequent days to detect a further decrease in platelet counts.

If suggestive **bleeding disorders** are present, there is no need to confirm the thrombocytopenia.

Hemorrhagic manifestations associated with thrombocytopenia:
- *petechiae*
- *ecchymoses*
- *epistaxis*
- *hemorrhagic bullae inside the mouth*
- *gingival bleeding*
- *excessive uterine bleeding*
- *conjunctival or retinal bleeding*

If there are no bleeding disorders, the existence of thrombocytopenia must be **confirmed** by ruling out pseudo-thrombocytopenia:

- repeat the platelet count with a different anticoagulant
- check blood film for decreased platelets and the absence of aggregates.

Pseudo thrombocytopenia
- *normal number of platelets in vivo*
- *but platelet aggregation in the test tube due to the anticoagulant (EDTA), which artificially lowers the platelet count given by the cell counters.*

Management

A risk of bleeding exists:

- if the platelet count is below 50 000/μL
- if bleeding time as measured by the Ivy technique is increased, *and* the platelet count is between 50 000 and 100 000/μL
- or if there is an associated risk factor, such as treatment with an anticoagulant or NSAID, peptic ulcer, severe hypertension, leiomyoma of the uterus, age >75 years.

If there is no risk of bleeding, withdrawal of drugs is decided upon on a case-by-case basis.

---

*Except for thrombocytopenia during treatment with heparin.

In the event of thrombocytopenia with risk of bleeding:

- Discontinue all medications not essential for life
- Search for signs of severity:
  - thrombocytopenia $< 50\,000/\mu L$
  - or hemorrhagic bullae inside the mouth
  - or retinal hemorrhages
  - or mucosal bleeding.

If one or more signs of a **severe** thrombocytopenia are present:

- The patient should be hospitalized
- Certain tests are urgently required
  - complete blood count
  - RBC phenotyping and tests for serum anti-RBC antibodies
  - search for a concomitant coagulation abnormality
  - bone marrow examination
- Emergency treatment must be instituted.

If no signs of severity are detected, close surveillance and consultation with a specialist are necessary.

Evidence implicating a drug in isolated thrombocytopenia*

The drug-related causes of thrombocytopenia are in the minority. Cases have been described with certain drugs belonging to most of the therapeutic classes.

Consider a drug-related etiology if one or more of the following criteria are present:

- The bone marrow is normal and rich in megakaryocytes.
- Thrombocytopenia develops in the month that follows institution of initial treatment with a drug or in the week after subsequent treatment with the drug.
- Thrombocytopenia resolves
  - fully
  - definitively
  - within 6 weeks of withdrawal of the medication
  - in the absence of symptomatic treatment (corticosteroids).

It confirms a drug-related etiology when: In vitro *tests for immunologic thrombocytopenia are positive.*
Principle: *demonstrate that the combined presence of patient's serum + drug (but not the drug or serum separately or the combined presence of a normal serum and the drug) produces platelet function changes or the binding of immunoglobulins to platelets.*
Procedure: *collect a serum specimen 3–5 days after discontinuation of the drug (the specimen may be frozen). A* **positive** *test result demonstrates the involvement of the drug; a* **negative** *result is inconclusive.*

---

*Without involvement of other blood cells, apart from possible hemorrhagic anemia.

- The **drug(s)** is (are) known to produce thrombocytopenia (refer to the information supplied by the manufacturer).

A drug-related etiology cannot be excluded because of the absence of one or more of these criteria.

Search for non drug-related causes:

- Central causes (aplasia, blood disorders), which can be ruled out by the results of the *bone marrow examination.*
- Other peripheral thrombocytopenias:
  - liver disease with or without hypersplenism (alcoholism)
  - bacterial and viral infections (HIV)
  - **idiopathic thrombocytopenic purpura (ITP), by far the most common cause of thrombocytopenia.**

Idiopathic thrombocytopenic purpura

Basis of a positive diagnosis of ITP:

- presence of platelet-associated immunoglobulins
- positive RBC Coombs test
- associated autoimmune disease (SLE) or presence of antinuclear antibodies
- persistence of thrombocytopenia more than 6 weeks after suspension of the drug
- delayed, slow and irregular response to corticosteroids
- recurrences on dosage reduction or on discontinuation of corticosteroids.

Antibodies attached to platelets
Principle: demonstration by various techniques (platelet Coombs test, ELISA) of immunoglobulins bound to the patient's platelets.
Interpretation:
- *positive:* suggests autoimmune thrombocytopenia but may also be positive at the acute phase of drug-induced thrombocytopenia
- *negative:* does not exclude autoimmune thrombocytopenia

Reference

Bénichou C, Solal-Céligny P. Standardization of definitions and criteria for causality assessment of adverse drug reactions. Drug-induced blood cytopenias. Report of an International Consensus Meeting. Nouv Rev Fh Hematol 1991; 33: 257–62.

Hackett T, Kelton JG, Powers P. Drug-induced platelet destruction. Seminars in Thrombosis and Hemostasis 1982; 8, no. 2.

Eosinophilia

Definition

Number of eosinophils $>450/\mu$L
$(0.45 \times 10^9/\text{L})$
   and
Percentage of eosinophils $>5\%$ of
leukocytes

This criterion is based on the need to exclude cases where an eosinophil count of more than 450/μL is accompanied by significant leukocytosis.

Criteria of severity

Eosinophilia is not severe *per se*, except in the context of a hypereosinophilic syndrome defined by eosinophilia in excess of 1500/μL lasting for more than 6 months. Aside from this exceptional situation, the severity of eosinophilia is related solely to the allergic manifestations that it accompanies:

- bronchospasm
- angioedema, urticaria
- liver injury
- acute nephropathy.

Evidence implicating a drug

Relating eosinophilia to a drug is difficult. The problem is further complicated by the possibility that a drug may aggravate a pre-existing eosinophilia, especially in the atopic patient.

- If eosinophilia is discovered in the absence of a previously known above normal increase in eosinophils, evidence for the following should be sought:
  - parasitic infestation
    - *youth*
    - *travel in countries where parasitic diseases are endemic*
    - *examine stools for parasite: if negative, repeat 4–6 weeks later (migration time of parasites in tissues)*
    - *serologic tests*
    - *in some cases, response to an anthelmintic treatment test*
  - atopic dermatitis or other pruritic skin disorder
  - nasopharyngeal and respiratory allergy
    - *allergic rhinitis*
    - *asthma*
    - *asthmatic cough*

However, one should note that drug-induced eosinophilia is more prevalent in atopic individuals.

- If it has been established that eosinophilia is of recent onset or has recently worsened, the same causes should be considered while giving greater credence to a drug-related origin, based on the following factors:
  - **time of onset**
    eosinophilia developed or became aggravated within 2–4 weeks of the start of the treatment
  - **reduction in eosinophilia** on discontinuation of the drug

    In atopic patients, this reduction may be incomplete: if no other measure is taken (e.g. stopping exposure to an allergen, use of corticosteroids), a reduction in the number of eosinophils of about 50% can be considered significant.

    The resolution of eosinophilia despite continued treatment does not disprove a possible relationship to the drug.

  - **associated signs**
    eosinophilia (or its aggravation) is accompanied by the onset or aggravation of other allergic signs known to occur with the drug or drugs
  - **elimination of the other causes** listed above.

Management

If no associated signs have occurred, eosinophilia is not a contraindication for continued drug treatment.

If one or more such signs have occurred, drug treatments initiated in the previous 4–8 weeks and which are not necessary for life should be discontinued.

Reintroduction of a medication may be contemplated only if the first episode is not accompanied by any allergic manifestation. A recurrence of eosinophilia suggests a relationship to the drug, though eosinophilia fluctuates in atopic individuals. For example, during a bacterial infection, it may disappear in the initial phase, reappear when the patient recovers and be mistakenly attributed to the treatment employed for the infection.

Hemolytic anemia

Drug-induced hemolytic anemia can involve four distinct mechanisms:
- The production—induced by drugs—of autoantibodies directed against red blood cells, causing **autoimmune hemolytic anemia.**
- The production of antidrug antibodies which, in some circumstances and after forming a complex with the drug, can bind to RBC and produce their lysis by complement activation. This is **immune hemolytic anemia.**
- Metabolic stress on constitutionally deficient red cells of individuals who have an **abnormality** of hemoglobin (methemoglobinemia) or of red blood cell enzymes (glucose-6-phosphate dehydrogenase—G6PD—deficiency).
- Hemolysis due to red cell fragmentation associated with intravascular microthrombi. This is **microangiopathic hemolytic anemia.**

Definition

Hemolytic anemia is characterized by:
- Anemia in which hemoglobin is less than
  12 g/dL in women
  13 g/dL in men

and with
- normal MCV

But pronounced reticulocytosis may result in a falsely increased MCV since the mean volume of the reticulocytes is larger than that of the erythrocytes.

and with
- marked reticulocytosis

But this does not occur when the process responsible also involves the precursors in the bone marrow (erythroblasts).

and with signs indicative of increased red blood cell destruction
  - **low levels of haptoglobin**
  - hyperbilirubinemia with marked predominance of unconjugated (indirect) bilirubin
  - increased levels of serum LDH
  - increased levels of serum iron

The most reliable sign
But it is not found at the initial stage of acute hemolysis.

Signs of severity

- Cardiovascular impact of anemia, which depends upon:
  - the hemoglobin level

Asthenia, dizziness, orthostatic hypotension, headache, tinnitus

    — the rapidity of onset of anemia

    — pre-existing cardiovascular   *Angina pectoris, heart failure*
      changes: age-related,
      atherosclerosis, etc.

- renal insufficiency   *Elevation of serum or plasma creatinin*

Evidence implicating a drug

The evidence depends largely on the
mechanism of hemolysis:

1. Autoimmune hemolytic anemia

- Gradual onset
- Positive direct Coombs test   *Detection of antibody attached to red cells*

- Demonstration of anti-red cell   ***Positive*** *tests confirm that the*
  antibodies   *hemolytic anemia is of autoimmune*
    — by indirect Coombs test   *origin*
    — by physical or chemical elution of   ***Negative*** *tests are inconclusive*
      antibodies bound to red cells,
      followed by indirect Coombs test

Drugs are a very rare cause ($< 10\%$) of autoimmune hemolytic anemia. Most autoimmune hemolytic anemias are idiopathic.

- Factors suggestive of a **drug-related**
  cause:
    — continuous administration for a   *At least four weeks*
      long period

    — dopamine agonist   *Especially alpha-methyldopa*
                                          Levodopa much more rarely

Any suspect drug must be withdrawn. On discontinuation of the drug, autoimmune hemolytic anemia abates very slowly, over several weeks or several months.

2. Immune hemolytic anemia

- **Abrupt** onset
    — back pain
    — fever
    — hypotension or shock
    — oliguria with very dark urine

- Severe anemia   *Hemoglobin $< 10\,g/dL$, often less*

- **Association with acute renal failure**   *This sign is of **great value** because its occurrence is exceptional in the other hemolytic anemias*

- Positive direct Coombs test   *However, anti-red cell antibodies are absent.*

Immune hemolytic anemia carries a high risk of mortality due to shock and/or acute renal failure. In all cases, **emergency hospitalization** in an intensive care unit is mandatory.

Virtually all immune hemolytic anemias are drug-related. The drug responsible can be identified by:

- Time sequence
  - drug taken less than 24 hours before the onset of the symptoms   *As a rule, the development of immune hemolytic anemia is biphasic:*
    - *sensitization with production of antibodies on initial administration of the drug*
    - *hemolysis triggered on subsequent administration*
- Laboratory studies
  - demonstration of **serum antibodies** directed against the drug or one of its metabolites   *Only a limited number of specialized laboratories are equipped to conduct tests for these antibodies. Tests may be performed on a frozen serum specimen after the acute episode is over.*

The drugs principally responsible for immune hemolytic anemia are listed in Table 1.

Table 1   Drugs implicated in cases of immune hemolytic anemia

Beta-lactam antibiotics	Rifampicin
Tetracyclines	Glafenine
Tolbutamide	Sulindac
Chlorpropamide	Ibuprofen
Quinine, quinidine	

Rechallenge with a drug whose involvement is confirmed or suspected is an absolute contraindication, because a recurrence is highly probable and often more serious.

3. Drug-induced hemolysis in a patient with an intrinsic red cell defect

- Ethnic origin: especially of Mediterranean ancestry
- Personal and family history of anemia, recurrent jaundice

- Abrupt onset
- Negative Coombs test
- Methemoglobinemia or enzyme deficiency

All oxidant drugs can precipitate a hemolytic crisis in these patients. The list of potentially hazardous drugs most commonly associated with G6PD deficiency (Table 2) must be reviewed to avoid relapses.

Table 2 Drugs that may cause hemolysis in individuals with G6PD deficiency

Acetanilide	Niridazole
Doxorubicin	Nitrofurantoin
Furazolidone	Phenazopyridine
Methylene blue	Primaquine
Nalidixic acid	Sulfamethoxazole

Source: After Beutler E. Glucose-6-phosphate deficiency. New England J Med 1991; 324: 169.

4. Microangiopathic hemolytic anemia

- May be associated with neurologic manifestations (convulsions, confusion, paresis) and renal failure
- Presence of a significant number of schistocytes, fragmented erythrocytes (examine the blood smear for evidence)
- Negative Coombs test
- Thrombocytopenia and/or disseminated intravascular coagulation

Several drugs can cause microangiopathic hemolytic anemia (Table 3), particularly oral contraceptives and some anticancer drugs (mitomycin C). Recovery on discontinuation of the drug is variable and slow.

Table 3 Drugs implicated in microangiopathic hemolytic anemia

Cancer chemotherapeutic agents	*Other drugs*
Mitomycin	Cyclosporin
Cisplatin	Oral contraceptives
Cytarabine	Metronidazole
Daunorubicin	Penicillamine
Lomustine	Penicillin

Source: After Kwaan HC. Miscellaneous secondary thrombotic micro-angiopathy. Semin Hematol 1987; 24: 141–6.

Reference

Habibi B, Solal-Céligny P, Bénichou C, et al. Anémies hémolytiques d'origine médicamenteuse. Résultets de réunions de consensus. Thérapie 1988; 43: 117–20.

BLOOD CYTOPENIA
DEFINITIONS

WHITE BLOOD CELLS

Neutropenia
Polynuclear neutrophils <1500/μL*

Severe neutropenia
Polynuclear neutrophils <500/μL*

Leukopenia (term to be used only in absence of differential blood count)
Leukocytes <3000/μL*

Agranulocytosis
Syndrome of sudden onset, with:
- severe neutropenia
- and the following clinical signs:
       fever
- **and** impaired general health
- **and** buccopharyngeal and/or perineal ulcers

*Figures given apply to white adults.

PLATELETS

Thrombocytopenia
Platelets <100 000/μL

If there are no hemorrhagic signs, the existence of thrombocytopenia must be confirmed by ruling out pseudothrombocytopenia:

- repeat the platelet count with a different anticoagulant;
- check blood film for decreased platelets and the absence of aggregates.

DEFICIENCY IN MORE THAN ONE BLOOD CELL LINE

If bone marrow data are unavailable, these terms are used:

Pancytopenia: or **Bicytopenia:**
Anemia (hemoglobin <10 g/dL)   Deficiency in two of the three blood cell lines
and Neutropenia
and Thrombocytoenia

If the results of a bone marrow biopsy (BMB) are available, these terms are used:

Pancytopenia (or bicytopenia) with normal marrow

Bone marrow aplasia
Pan- (or bi-) cytopenia
and BMB showing hypocellular marrow
and no infiltration
and no fibrosis

If the data are based only on a bone marrow aspirate (BMA), the term used is:

Probable bone marrow aplasia
Pan- (or bi-) cytopenia
and BMB showing hypocellular marrow
and no infiltration

NEUTROPENIA
CHRONOLOGICAL CRITERIA

Time to onset of the reaction		Very suggestive	Suggestive	Compatible	Inconclusive	Incompatible	
				From start of drug administration	*From end of drug administration*	*With regard to start of drug administration*	*From end of drug administration*
	Initial treatment			Any time interval while on drug	Occurrence within 30 days or Discovery after 30 days	Drug taken before the onset of the reaction	Occurrence after 30 days
	Subsequent treatment with or without previous history in relation to the same drug		*From start of drug administration* ≤7 days	*From start of drug administration* >7 days			

Course of the reaction		Very suggestive	Suggestive	Compatible	Inconclusive	Not suggestive
	Without stopping the drug			Continuing decrease in neutrophil counts		
	After stopping the drug		Neutrophils >1500 within 30 days		Return of the neutrophil count to the normal range	
					Neutrophils ≤1500 after 30 days	

THROMBOCYTOPENIA
CHRONOLOGICAL CRITERIA

		Very suggestive	Suggestive	Compatible	Inconclusive	Incompatible
Time to onset of the reaction	Initial treatment		*From start of drug administration* ≤1 month	*From start of drug administration* >1 month	*From end of drug administration* Occurrence within 30 days or Discovery after 30 days	*With regard to start of drug administration* Drug taken after the onset of the reaction
	Subsequent treatment with or without previous history in relation to the same drug	*From start of drug administration* ≤7 days	*From start of drug administration* 8–30 days			*From end of drug administration* Occurrence after 30 days

		Very suggestive	Suggestive	Compatible	Inconclusive	Not suggestive
Course of the reaction	Without stopping the drug			Continuing decrease in platelet counts	No recovery of thrombocytopenia	
	After stopping the drug			Recovery within 3 weeks (with or without corticosteroids)	Recovery after 3 weeks (with or without corticosteroids)	Relapse of thrombocytopenia after 3 weeks

APLASTIC ANEMIA
CHRONOLOGICAL CRITERIA

		Compatible	Incompatible
Time to onset from the start of the drug administration	Initial treatment	>4 days	Reaction occurred before the 4th day of treatment
	Subsequent treatment	All time intervals	Reaction occurred before starting the drug

	Compatible	Incompatible
Time to onset from the end of the drug administration	≤120 days	>120 days

		Compatible	Inconclusive	Incompatible
Course of the reaction	Without stopping the drug		No change or Aggravation	Improvement in pancytopenia or bicytopenia
	After stopping the drug	Spontaneous recovery within 6 months: neutrophils >1500 and platelets >100 000	No change or Aggravation or Improvement with supportive therapy	

DRUG-INDUCED ACUTE IMMUNE HEMOLYTIC ANEMIA
DEFINITIONS

Anemia	Hemoglobin <10 g/dL
Acute	Developing in less than 24 hours
Hemolytic	Presence of two of these three criteria: • clinical: fever, back pain, chills, headache, vomiting, shock • hemoglobinuria • hyperbilirubinemia or reticulocytosis or reduced serum haptoglobin level
Immune hemolytic	Hemolysis induced by antidrug antibody in the serum

ACUTE AUTOIMMUNE HEMOLYTIC ANEMIA
CHRONOLOGICAL CRITERIA

Time to onset of the reaction	Very suggestive	Suggestive	Compatible	Inconclusive	Incompatible
Initial treatment			*From start of drug administration* >15 days		*With regard to start of drug administration* Reaction occurred before the 15th day unless antidrug antibodies are present in the serum
Subsequent treatment with or without previous history in relation to the same drug	*From start of drug administration* ≤1 day				*From end of drug administration* First symptoms after 1 day

Course of the reaction	Very suggestive	Suggestive	Compatible	Inconclusive	Not suggestive
Without stopping the drug		Aggravation of clinical signs or laboratory abnormalities		Persistence of laboratory abnormalities or no information on the course	Improvement of laboratory abnormalities
After stopping the drug		Regression of the laboratory abnormalities within 15 days		No information on the course	No change or aggravation of laboratory abnormalities after 15 days

3 Cutaneous reactions

Jean-Claude Roujeau

General information

Skin disorders are the most common adverse reactions attributed to drugs. About 5% of hospitalizations in dermatology departments are attributed to them. Any skin disorder can be imitated, induced or aggravated by drugs. With rare exceptions, drug-induced skin disorders have little symptomatic specificity, if any at all.

Severe reactions (involving hospitalization, and even life-threatening in some cases) account for less than 10% of all skin disorders due to drugs that bring the patient to a hospital consultation. The most common ones, pruritus, maculopapular eruptions and urticaria, account for about 80% of all drug-related skin reactions.

On the whole, little is known about the pathophysiologic mechanisms of drug-induced dermatitis. They are usually considered to be hypersensitivity reactions, but this has actually been demonstrated only with a few particular reactions and a few drugs (urticaria and Type I anaphylactic reaction to penicillins, mediated by IgE antibodies).

Reference

Bigby M, Jick S, Jick H, Arndt K. Drug-induced cutaneous reactions. A report from the Boston Collaborative Drug Surveillance program on 154 538 consecutive inpatients, 1975 to 1982. JAMA 1986; 256: 3358–63.

Adverse Drug Reactions. A Practical Guide to Diagnosis and Management. Edited by C. Bénichou.
©1994 John Wiley & Sons Ltd.

Urticaria

Definition

The common form of urticaria is an eruption consisting of pruritic edematous wheals, which may spread, and evanescent papules (lasting from a few minutes to a few hours). The papules are barely erythematous, just bordering on the color of normal skin. The course is recurrent. Chronic urticaria is defined by recurrent episodes over a period of more than 6 weeks.

This involves edema of the superficial portion of the dermis, secondary to increased vascular permeability via the effect of multiple inflammatory response mediators released by mast cells.

Other forms

Two forms should be distinguished from common urticaria:

- **fixed urticaria** due to vasculitis, notably during the course of serum sickness
- **deep urticaria**: angioedema affecting different sites, including the face and mucous membranes.

Signs of severity

Urticaria can be **severe** either because of its **localization** (angioedema of the upper airways) or because of its **association** with systemic anaphylactic symptoms.

Etiology

Urticaria is extremely common. Drugs are not responsible for more than 5–10% of the cases, in either the acute or the chronic forms.

The agents most often responsible for the acute forms include iodinated contrast media, blood products, vaccines or sera, general or local

The etiology remains unclear in more than half the cases of urticaria. In acute urticaria, investigation should be directed towards:

- *a reaction to a food allergen*
- *an acute parasitic or viral infection.*

anesthetics, beta-lactam antibiotics, enzymes, opiates, sulfonamides, barbiturates, glafenine.

A drug-related etiology is much more difficult to demonstrate in chronic urticaria. Inquiries should concentrate on colorants (especially, but not exclusively, tartrazine) and aspirin (with potential crossreactivity with all NSAIDs).

The most frequent causes of chronic urticaria are:

- *physical factors (pressure, cold, etc.)*
- *certain autoimmune diseases*
- *localized infections.*

Evidence implicating a drug

When acute urticaria is drug-induced, the very suggestive time of onset, from less than an hour to a few hours after administration of the drug, generally makes the cause obvious.

The onset is very different in fixed urticaria related to serum sickness, where the wheals appear 6–12 days after initiation of the treatment.

Management

Discontinue the administration of drugs instituted recently, provided that their sudden withdrawal is not considered dangerous.

The administration of **H₁-receptor antagonists** (**H₁ antihistamines**) orally or intramuscularly is always recommended.

H₁ antihistaminic drugs are not very effective on existing lesions, but they can prevent immediate recurrences.

Oral or injectable corticosteroids should be avoided in mild eruptions. In the more severe forms of urticaria (involving the deeper layers of the mucous membranes and endangering respiratory function, or those associated with anaphylactic shock), emergency treatment consists of **epinephrine** injected subcutaneously or intramuscularly.

The reintroduction of a drug suspected of having induced acute urticaria should be avoided. When its use is imperative, preventive measures *must* be taken.

For general anesthetics, iodinated contrast media or blood products, one can use as prevention H₁ and H₂ antihistamines and corticosteroids in injectable form.

In penicillin-induced urticaria, the risk of crossreactivity with another beta-lactam antibiotic is estimated to be between 10 and 20%. Therefore, an antibiotic of a different class should be used when possible.

If the use of a beta-lactam antibiotic is imperative (and only in this case), skin tests should be performed: prick tests, followed, if negative, by intradermal tests. There is no risk in using penicillins if the skin tests are negative to the major and different minor antigens. If one test is positive, the hazard of a severe anaphylactic reaction is so great that treatment should not be considered without prior desensitization.

Several methods of desensitization have been published and have shown satisfactory results.

Diffuse maculopapular erythematous eruptions

Definition

The lesions consist of small fixed erythematous spots (macules); the spots, measuring a few millimeters in diameter, are sometimes slightly infiltrated (maculopapules), appearing within days or hours over an extensive part of the body, starting at the head and descending and disappearing in 2 to 10 days, with or without fine desquamation. They are nearly always accompanied by pruritus. The mucous membranes are usually spared.

Different forms are described:

- *morbilliform* eruption, when the macules are clearly visible and well-defined
- *roseolar* eruption, when the macules are very pale and barely visible
- *scarlatiniform* eruption, when the lesions are confluent and form large patches of continuous erythema.

Signs of severity

Hospitalization is mandatory when the lesions are confluent with secondary evolution to erythroderma or when mucous membranes are involved, especially if the lesions are erosive.

Etiology

The part played by drugs in the etiology of this disorder is quite different in adults and in children. In adults, drug reactions are the most frequent cause of maculopapular eruptions. In children, the leading causes are infections, especially viral.

For many drugs, figures are available on the incidence of maculopapular eruptions in patients taking them:

- 10% or more for gold salts
- 3–5% for aminopenicillins
- 3–4% for sulfonamides
- approximately 2% for the other

In children and infants, the following should be ruled out:

- if the patient presents with a morbilliform or roseolar eruption
  - measles
  - rubella
  - exanthema subitum

beta-lactams, allopurinol and blood products
- 1–2% for H_2 antihistamines, angiotensine converting enzyme inhibitors and most NSAIDs.

Iodinated contrast media and general anesthetics may also produce maculopapular rashes but more rarely than urticaria.

- *erythema infectiosum*
- *if the patient presents with a scarlatiniform eruption*
  - *Kawasaki disease*
  - *scarlet fever*

In adults, the following should be considered:

- *if the patient presents with a morbilliform or roseolar eruption*
  - *infectious mononucleosis*
  - *reactivation of a cytomegalovirus infection*
  - *hepatitis B viral infection*
  - *rickettsia*
  - *secondary syphilis*
  - *primary HIV infection*
- *if the patient presents with a scarlatiniform eruption*
  - *toxic shock syndrome due to staphylococci*

Management

The possibility of evolution to erythroderma or, more exceptionally, to toxic epidermal necrolysis, justifies withdrawing the suspect drugs (if this poses no immediate danger). It has not been demonstrated conclusively that stopping the drugs will actually affect the evolution of the lesions.

It is desirable to investigate the possibility of a viral infection (history of contacts, serologic tests at a 2-week interval), especially in children.

The administration of H_1 antihistamine drugs has little effect on the course of the eruption but may help to relieve pruritus if the itching is troublesome.

The administration of systemic corticosteroids has not been proved effective in this type of cutaneous reaction.

Rechallenge should be avoided because it could cause a more severe reaction than occurred initially.

No diagnostic test has proved to be of value in this type of eruption.

Evidence implicating a drug

Timing

Maculopapular eruptions usually appear 5–10 days after the start of the treatment, sometimes after its discontinuation in the case of short treatment.

Any shorter or longer time sequence is compatible.

Symptoms

Symptoms are diagnostically unhelpful.

A severe pruritus and polymorphous lesions (purpura-like appearance of the center of certain macules, urticarial papules, rather indistinct "target" lesions) tend to point to a drug-induced origin.

Very high fever, enanthemata or multiple lymph node enlargement suggest a viral etiology.

Predisposing factors

Infectious mononucleosis, HIV infection, active cytomegalovirus infections or chronic lymphocytic leukemia will predispose to drug-induced maculopapular eruptions.

For example, cutaneous reactions to aminopenicillins are more frequent during infectious mononucleosis (70–100%), but this is not necessarily an "allergy to penicillins".

Erythroderma

Definition

This term, which refers to a serious condition, should not be used for any extensive erythema but should be reserved for a disorder that fulfils precise criteria.

The lesions involve the **entire skin surface** (with the possible exception of a few "spared intervals" of healthy skin). The skin is **thickened, infiltrated, erythematous, oozing** or **scaling**.

The palms and soles are usually affected by hyperkeratosis with frequent fissuring. The mucous membranes are spared. Pruritus is unremitting, severe and often causes insomnia.

The onset of the lesions is progressive, over a period of several days or even weeks.

The course is of long duration.

The temperature is often moderately elevated: 38–38.5°C. **Lymphadenopathy** is a usual occurrence, and the nodes may be greatly enlarged. Leukocytosis is frequently observed, with eosinophilia which can be considerable.

Signs of severity

Erythroderma is always a serious disorder that necessitates hospitalization. It may be life-threatening in patients who tolerate poorly the systemic effects (loss of water and electrolytes, loss of calories), especially aged patients or those with heart failure.

Etiology

Cutaneous adverse reactions to drugs account for approximately 5–10% of the cases of erythroderma, far behind the number associated with contact dermatitis and psoriasis.

While there are many non drug-related causes, it is predominantly associated with three diseases:

- *contact dermatitis*
- *psoriasis*
- *epidermotropic T cell lymphoma.*

The principal offenders in drug-induced erythroderma are:

- anticonvulsants, notably phenytoin and carbamazepine
- sulfasalazine
- antibacterial sulfonamides
- pyrazolone derivatives
- gold salts
- penicillins.

Lastly, over 50% of erythroderma cases are idiopathic. Some will evolve to T-cell lymphoma over a course of several months or years.

Evidence implicating a drug

Timing of onset

The most suggestive timing is from 2–4 weeks after introduction of the drug.

Shorter or longer time sequences are still compatible.

Signs

The absence of a history of psoriasis, a rapid onset or lesions starting in an area exposed to light (face, back of the hands) are evidence pointing to a drug-related cause.

The presence of greatly enlarged lymph nodes suggestive of lymphoma is not conclusive evidence against a drug-related etiology.

Further examination

Histologic examination of the skin is absolutely essential.

The appearance may be specific to psoriasis, contact dermatitis or lymphoma, or it may remain nonspecific (adverse reactions to drugs or other etiology).

Management

Any treatment whose abrupt withdrawal is not dangerous should be discontinued. Patients with erythroderma should be hospitalized for an etiologic evaluation and symptomatic or etiologic treatment should be started.

Vascular purpura

Definition

The lesions consist of infiltrated, palpable petechiae predominating on the lower extremities. There are no ecchymoses or signs of bleeding. The platelets are quantitatively and qualitatively normal.

This purpura results from inflammatory lesions of the blood vessels in the superficial portion of the dermis.

Other skin lesions may be associated with the purpura:

- hemorrhagic bullae
- small, round dermal nodules
- urticarial papules
- punched-out cutaneous necrosis.

Pathology of the lesions

The most typical picture is leukocytoclastic vasculitis, combining fibrinoid necrosis of capillary walls and a perivascular infiltrate consisting of damaged polymorphonuclear neutrophils.

Signs of severity

The purpura may be an isolated manifestation or it may be associated with joint and muscle pain or with extremely serious systemic conditions: peripheral neuropathy, glomerulopathy, intestinal bleeding and/or intussception.

Etiology

In the largest series of cases reported, drugs account for less than 10% of the cases.

The possible causes of vascular purpura are very numerous: 30–50% of cases are termed idiopathic.

Dozens of cases of vascular purpura attributed to drugs have been reported in the literature but a medicine's implication often appears

Vascular purpura may be classified as follows:

- **Purpura secondary** to bacterial infection (meningococcemia, gonococcemia, bacterial endocarditis, focus of localized infection etc.), to viral infection (hepatitis B, etc.), or to neoplasia (especially lymphoproliferative disorders).
- Purpura associated with an abnormal immunologic response (**immunologic purpura**). This is seen in cryoglobulinemia, Sjögren's syndrome, rheumatoid arthritis, systemic lupus erythematosus, etc.
- **Henoch–Schönlein purpura** deserves separate consideration because of its occurrence in children, its usual association with other symptoms and the deposit of IgA in skin capillaries.
- Purpura may be the presenting symptom of certain types of **systemic vasculitis** (such as polyarteritis nodosa, Wegener's granulomatosis, etc.).

doubtful. The agents incriminated most often are:

- *antibacterial sulfonamides*
- *pyrazole derivatives*
- *hydantoins*
- *thiourea derivatives*
- *penicillins.*

In practice, acute purpura is usually secondary to an infection, while chronic relapsing purpura is usually seen in immunologic purpura.

Evidence implicating a drug

The most suggestive time to onset is 7–21 days in cases where a new drug is administered for the first time.

Other times to onset are compatible.

Management

Febrile acute purpura of recent onset necessitates emergency hospitalization after an aminopenicillin injection is administered to protect against the possibility of meningococcemia.

In the other cases, an etiologic evaluation is necessary. Suspect drugs whose withdrawal is not considered dangerous must be discontinued.

Reference

Guillaume JC, Roujeau JC, Chevrant-Breton J, et al. Comment imputer un accident cutané à un médicament. Application aux purpuras vasculaires. (How to relate an adverse cutaneous reaction to a drug. Application to vascular purpura.) Ann Dermatol Venereol 1987; 114: 721–4.

VASCULAR PURPURA
DEFINITION

The diagnosis of vascular purpura can be accepted in three circumstances:

- purpura diagnosed clinically **and**
  - either a normal platelet count ($> 100\,000/\mu L$)
  - or histologic signs of vasculitis localized to the skin:
    most commonly leukocytoclastic and/or necrotizing but all histologic features of vasculitis are acceptable
  - or palpable and/or "polymorphic" clinical features (e.g. necrotic, ulcerated, pustular purpura).

VASCULAR PURPURA
CHRONOLOGICAL CRITERIA

		Very suggestive	Suggestive	Compatible	Inconclusive	Incompatible	
						With regard to start of drug administration	After stopping the drug*
Time to onset of the reaction	Initial treatment	From start of drug administration 7-21 days		From start of drug administration <7 days or >21 days			≥21 days
	Subsequent treatment without previous history			From start of drug administration All time intervals		Drug taken after the onset of the reaction	
	Subsequent treatment with previous history in relation to the same drug	From start of drug administration ≤3 days		From start of drug administration >3 days			

*No time interval can be considered as incompatible if the drug and/or its metabolites are still present in the body at the time the reaction occurs.

		Very suggestive	Suggestive	Compatible	Inconclusive	Incompatible
Course of the reaction	Without stopping the drug		Aggravation or New flare		Improvement or Unknown course	Complete resolution
	After stopping the drug*		Subsidence of the skin or visceral disorders without symptomatic treatment within 21 days		Improvement due to symptomatic treatment or Precocious death or Unknown course	New flare or Spread of the lesions

*Taking into account the time necessary for its elimination from the body.

Drug-induced photosensitivity

Definition

Photosensitivity refers to exaggerated and/or abnormal responses to light.

It is classified into phototoxic reactions (by far the most common) caused by the direct effect of the absorption of light energy by the drug, and photoallergic reactions that involve an immunologic response.

Typically, it presents as a "sunburn" limited to areas exposed to light (face, neck, back of hands).

Clinical appearance

- Bullae over the hands or feet
- Photo-onycholysis (nail plate detachment at its distal and lateral extremities)
- Intense pigmentation of areas exposed to light
- Polymorphic eczematiform and pseudo-urticarial lesions extending beyond the sunlight-exposed areas in photoallergic cases.

Etiology

A drug-related cause should be suspected in recent photosensitivity with no past history of occurrence.

Non drug-related causes include:

- *certain congenital dermatoses with photosensitivity*
- *porphyria*
- *lupus erythematosus*
- *polymorphous light eruption*
- *contact-induced photosensitivity (plants, perfumes, cosmetics, etc.).*

Among the very large number of offending drugs, the most common are:

- amiodarone
- tetracyclines
- phenothiazines
- thiazides
- sulfonamides
- griseofulvin
- quinolones.

Evidence implicating a drug

All temporal relationships are compatible with phototoxicity, bearing in mind that two factors are involved: administration of a drug and exposure to sunlight.

In photoallergy, there has to be a minimum interval of 5 days between the time that the drug is first taken and the occurrence of the reaction to establish a drug-induced photoallergic response (in cases of first administration).

Management

In most cases, the disorders can be corrected simply by avoiding sunlight exposure. If this can be done, the drug need not be withdrawn.

Extensive skin detachment forming an actual burn is exceptional but may occur and will require hospitalization.

References

Epstein JH, Wintroub BU. Photosensitivity due to drugs. Drugs 1985; 30: 42–57.

Roujeau JC, Beani JC, Dubertret L, et al. Photosensibilité cutanée médicamenteuse. Résultats d'une réunion de consensus. Thérapie 1989; 44: 223–7.

CUTANEOUS PHOTOSENSITIVITY
DEFINITIONS

This term refers to exaggerated and/or abnormal cutaneous reactions to sunlight.

This possibility should be considered in a patient taking **medicine** who has an eruption occurring predominantly **in exposed areas** (face, neck, hands or feet) following **exposure to sunlight**. A distinction is usually made between two mechanisms, based on evidence pointing to:

Phototoxicity	Photoallergy
• early onset • lesions well limited to areas exposed to sunlight • monomorphic appearance of severe sunburn • subsides on avoidance of sunlight exposure, with or without withdrawal of the drug • subsides on withdrawal of the drug, with or without avoidance of sunlight exposure • histological lesions: erythema caused by light exposure, unicellular necrosis ("sunburn cells")	• onset after more than 5 days of exposure to sunlight and to the drug, when given for the first time • extension beyond sunlight-exposed areas • polymorphic appearance, often eczematiform • subsides slowly after withdrawal of the drug • histologic lesions: similar to those of contact dermatitis with spongiosis and exocytosis

DRUG-INDUCED PHOTOTOXICITY
CHRONOLOGICAL CRITERIA

		Very suggestive	Suggestive	Compatible	Inconclusive	Incompatible
Time to onset of the reaction	With regard to start of drug administration			From start of drug administration		After stopping the drug*
	Drug taken after the onset of the reaction			All time intervals while on drug		All time intervals

*After the time necessary for the drug to be cleared from the body.

		Very suggestive	Suggestive	Compatible	Inconclusive	Not suggestive
Course of the reaction	Without stopping the drug		Aggravation with exposure to UVA		Absence of exposure to UVA	Improvement despite exposure to UVA
	After cessation of the drug*		Improvement with exposure to UVA		Improvement in the absence of exposure to UVA	Aggravation whatever the exposure to UVA

*Taking into account the time necessary for its elimination from the body.

DRUG-INDUCED PHOTOALLERGY
CHRONOLOGICAL CRITERIA

		Very suggestive	Suggestive	Compatible	Inconclusive	Incompatible	After stopping the drug*
Time to onset of the reaction	Initial treatment			From start of drug administration ≥5 days		From start of drug administration <5 days	≥21 days
	Subsequent treatment without previous history			From start of drug administration ≥3 hours		From start of drug administration <3 hours	
	Subsequent treatment with previous history in relation to the same drug	From start of drug administration 3–72 hours		From start of drug administration >3 days			

*No time interval can be considered as incompatible if the drug and/or its metabolites are still present in the body at the time the reaction occurs.

		Very suggestive	Suggestive	Compatible	Inconclusive	Incompatible
Course of the reaction	Without stopping the drug		Aggravation with exposure to UVA		Absence of exposure to UVA	Improvement despite exposure to UVA
	After stopping the drug*		Improvement despite exposure to UVA		Absence of exposure to UVA or Aggravation despite exposure to UVA	

*Taking into account the time necessary for its elimination from the body.

Bullous eruptions

Bullae are circumscribed, elevated lesions, containing fluid, that are larger than 5 mm (when smaller than 5 mm, they are called vesicles).

Bullous diseases are rare. Limited lesions call for rapid consultation with a specialist, while extensive lesions demand emergency hospitalization. The disease is potentially life-threatening. Precise diagnosis usually requires histologic examination of a skin biopsy. Drug-induced bullous lesions may have a number of clinical features.

Erythema multiforme and Stevens–Johnson syndrome

Definition

The definition (purely clinical) is based on the appearance of the primary lesion.

Target or iris lesion

This is a round lesion of variable size (usually 0.5–2 cm), which includes, from the periphery to the center, an erythematous border, an edematous ring, and a darker or purpuric center that may become bullous.

The lesions, all identical in appearance, number from a few dozen to hundreds and predominate on the extensor surfaces of the extremities.

Erosive mucosal lesions may be observed in about one-third of the cases.

The course is favorable and self-limiting in 10–20 days.

Drug-induced lesions are often atypical, varying in size, with an irregular outline and the intermediate edematous ring is often absent.

Clinical forms

Cases characterized by severe mucosal lesions accompanied by bullous skin lesions are called Stevens–Johnson syndrome.

Signs of severity

Severe complications are uncommon. They consist of erosive mucosal lesions, affecting the eyes in particular, that may leave severe irreversible sequelae.

Etiology

There are many causes of erythema multiforme and Stevens–Johnson syndrome: more than 100 different causes have been reported. Approximately one-third of the cases are idiopathic, one-third are caused by drugs and one-third are secondary to infections.

The list of drugs implicated in at least one case of erythema multiforme or Stevens–Johnson syndrome is extremely long. The agents most often responsible include:

- antibacterial sulfonamides
- barbiturates and other antiepileptic drugs (carbamazepine, phenytoin)
- beta-lactam antibiotics
- NSAIDs.

Among the infectious causes of erythema multiforme or Stevens–Johnson syndrome, two are far more frequent than the others:

- *recurrent herpes*
- *Mycoplasma pneumoniae infections.*

Evidence implicating a drug

Timing

The suggestive time sequence is 1–3 weeks after the introduction of a new drug.

Other timings are compatible.

Symptoms

Target lesions are mostly atypical in a drug-induced reaction.

The more the target lesions are typical, the more they suggest an infectious origin.

Management

Emergency hospitalization is required for any patient presenting with severe erythema multiforme as manifested by extensive skin lesions and/or by mucosal lesions.

Toxic epidermal necrosis (Lyell's syndrome)

Definition

Toxic epidermal necrosis (TEN) is the most spectacular and most severe form of bullous dermatosis.

It usually begins as an atypical erythema multiforme with lesions that spread rapidly and become confluent, whereupon the epidermis comes off in large sheets, resembling an extensive burn.

The slightest trauma peels off the epidermis, leaving a bright red, oozing, denuded dermis.

There are severe erosive mucosal lesions similar in appearance to those seen in Stevens–Johnson syndrome.

Regeneration of the epidermis takes approximately 3 weeks, during which time the patient is at risk of severe complications, notably of an infective nature. Sequelae, especially involving the eyes, are a frequent occurrence.

Histology

Skin biopsy reveals detachment at the epidermal-dermal junction with necrosis of the full thickness of the epidermis.

Biopsy makes it possible to exclude the diagnosis of staphylococcal scalded skin syndrome (SSSS), also called Ritter-Lyell syndrome, typically seen in young children and where the separation is more superficial and occurs under the horny layer (stratum corneum) of the skin.

Signs of severity

The mortality rate in TEN exceeds 20%. Extensive lesions and old age are adverse prognostic factors.

Etiology

No nondrug etiology has yet been established for TEN.

However:

- *in 5% of cases, no drug had been taken by the patient in the days preceding the reaction.*
- *In one-third of cases, the involvement of drugs appears doubtful.*

The list of drugs incriminated is very long. The agents most often responsible are the same as in Stevens–Johnson syndrome:

- antibacterial sulfonamides
- barbiturates and other antiepileptic drugs (carbamazepine, phenytoin)
- beta-lactam antibiotics
- NSAIDs.

Evidence implicating a drug

The suspect drugs are those introduced recently. The most characteristic time to onset is 1–3 weeks.

In the case of a drug that has not been administered previously, it is believed that a time interval of less than 24 hours is not compatible with the causation of TEN.

Management

In the event of a bullous eruption suggesting the beginning of TEN, it is mandatory that the administration of all suspect drugs be stopped and that emergency hospitalization of the patient be ordered in a specialized department.

If the involvement is already severe, an intravenous infusion of isotonic solution should be started before the patient is transferred.

Refrain from administering corticosteroids, which have no effect on the course of the disease but will simply worsen the prognosis by enhancing infective complications.

Reference

Roujeau JC, Chosidow O, Saïag Ph, Guillaume JC. Toxic epidermal necrolysis (Lyell Syndrome). J Am Acad Dermatol 1990; 23: 1039–58.

Fixed drug eruptions

Definition

These consist of one or more quite large (1–10 cm in diameter) round, inflammatory, erythematous and pruritic lesions that appear within a few hours after ingestion of the causative drug.

This erythema, accompanied by a burning sensation, may in some cases be followed by a bullous eruption. The erythema subsides in a few days, leaving a grayish or slate-colored pigmentation.

The mucous membranes of the mouth and genitals may be affected, usually through the extension of the skin lesion adjacent to the mucosal area.

Rechallenge produces, within a few hours, a return of the inflammatory reaction (which may be accompanied by bullae) on the original pigmented area, sometimes with the appearance of one or more new lesions.

Signs of severity

Exceptionally, the progressive extension of the number and size of the lesions during recurrences may lead to a severe bullous skin eruption.

Etiology

This is one of the few dermatoses specifically caused by drugs. There is no other known cause.

More than 100 drugs have been implicated. The ones most often responsible are:

- phenacetin
- phenolphthalein
- barbiturates
- certain tetracyclines
- sulfonamides.

Management

In exceptional cases with extensive lesions, emergency hospitalization is necessary.

For localized forms, only the use of topical antiseptics is justified while waiting for the lesions to heal.

The patient should be cautioned about the risk of a more severe relapse if the suspect drug is readministered.

Evidence implicating a drug

Timing

In practice, the disorder is always diagnosed at the time of a recurrence. The highly suggestive timing between the administration of the drug and the onset of the eruption is a few hours (less than 24 hours).

It is still compatible up to 72 hours.

Reference

Kauppinen K, Stubb S. Fixed eruptions: causative drugs and challenge tests. Brit J Dermatol 1985; 112: 575–8.

Acute generalized exanthematous pustulosis (AGEP)

Definition

This term refers to an acute febrile eruption consisting of a very large number of milky micropustules developing on an inflammatory erythema. The lesions start on the face or in the main skin creases and extend in a few days. They are sometimes accompanied by considerable granulocytosis. The pustules are sterile. The eruption disappears in 8–10 days.

Pustular psoriasis: lesions identical to those of AGEP, but of slower onset and with a more prolonged evolution, may develop in patients with psoriasis, often as a result of a therapeutic error.

Other appearances
In about a quarter of cases, other skin lesions are associated with the pustules (purpura, vesicles, atypical target lesions similar to those of erythema multiforme).

Etiology

If we exclude pustular psoriasis, 60–80% of AGEP cases appear to be caused by drugs.

Antibiotics (aminopenicillin and macrolides) are by far the most common offenders.

Exanthematous pustular dermatitis can be caused by a reaction to mercury (contact with the skin, inhalation or ingestion) and by enteroviral infections (coxsackie virus, echo virus).

Evidence implicating a drug

Timing

In pustular eruptions attributed to antibiotics, the interval between the administration of the drug and the eruption is less than 48 hours, sometimes only a few hours.

Management

Discontinue exposure to the causative drug. The clinical features are usually severe enough to justify hospitalization.

Readministration of the causative agent carries a high risk of recurrence.

Reference

Roujeau JC, Bioulac-Sage P, Bourseau C, et al. Acute generalized exanthematous pustulosis. Analysis of 63 cases. Arch Dermatol 1991; 127: 1333–8

BULLOUS ERUPTIONS

	Erythema multiforme	Stevens–Johnson syndrome	Toxic epidermal necrolysis	Fixed drug eruption	Acute generalized exanthematic pustulosis	Bullous pemphigoid	Pemphigus	Porphyria cutanea tarda
Age	Adolescent young adult	Any age	Any age	Any age	Any age	Elderly	40–50 years	40–50 years Alcoholism
Pattern and distribution of bullae	Typical targets Limbs	Atypical targets Widespread	Detachment of large epidermal sheets	One to few large bullae	Pustules widespread/main folds	Tense bullae widespread Pruritus	Flaccid bullae Chest	Erosions on the hands± face
Nikolsky's sign	–	–	+	–	–	–	+	–
Mucous membrane involvement	–	++	++	±	Rare	Rare	+P. vulgaris (PV) –P. foliaceous (PF)	–
Location of the split on pathology	Basement membrane zone (BMZ)				Intra-epidermal subcorneal	Basement membrane zone	Intra-epidermal (PV) Subcorneal (PF)	Basement membrane zone
Skin immunofluorescence	–	–	–	–	–	+linear	+network	–
Anti-epidermis antibodies	–	–	–	–	–	+anti-BMZ	+anti-epidermal cell surface	–
Proportion of drug-related cases	<30%	~30%	60–90%	~100%	60–80%	?rare	~10%	Non-exceptional (triggering)
Drugs	Antimicrobial sulfonamides Anticonvulsants beta-lactam antibiotics NSAIDs			Phenacetin Amidopyrine Phenolphthalein Barbiturates Tetracyclines Sulfonamides	Amino-penicillins Macrolides	Penicillins Amiodarone Furosemide	Sulfhydrilated drugs D-penicillamine Pyritinol Tiopronine Captopril	Chloroquine Hydroxy-chloroquine Busulfan Oestrogens Androgens etc.

4 Anaphylactic and anaphylactoid reactions

Christian Bénichou

Anaphylactic reactions

Anaphylactic shock

Shock is an acute circulatory failure marked by a fall in blood pressure (systolic BP < 70 mmHg) and a small, rapid or unobtainable pulse. The term anaphylactic should be reserved for those with an allergic mechanism.

An anaphylactic reaction is a result of the liberation of endogenous chemical mediators released following the reaction between IgE antibodies (situated at the cell surface) and an antigen that has been reintroduced (second contact).

The term anaphylactoid is used to refer to reactions, generally drug-induced, that reflect the liberation of the same chemical mediators without the intervention of IgE antibodies.

Anaphylactic shock is characterized by the abrupt onset of a severe general malaise, with chills and sensation of imminent death, pruritus of the extremities, pallor or, in contrast, generalized flushing, followed by sweating. Sometimes, a state of torpor sets in that may go as far as loss of consciousness with hypothermia.

- Other signs of shock are:
  - **gastrointestinal signs**: vomiting and diarrhea

*The presence of signs of allergy (urticaria, angioedema, rash, asthma-like dyspnea) is evidence of anaphylactic shock and makes it possible to distinguish it from **cardiogenic shock** (acute insufficient ventricular filling or ejection) and **hypovolemic shock** (with decreased circulating blood volume).*

If the patient has tachycardia, you may rule out a vasovagal syncope, which is characterized by bradycardia.

Adverse Drug Reactions. A Practical Guide to Diagnosis and Management. Edited by C. Bénichou.
©1994 John Wiley & Sons Ltd.

- **pulmonary signs**: rapid, shallow respiration or asthma-like paroxysmal obstructive dyspnea
- **neurological signs**: convulsions or coma
- The shock may be accompanied by
  - **mucocutaneous signs**: urticaria, angioedema, frequent itching of the extremities or the tongue.

Less severe forms

- Less severe systemic reactions: fall in blood pressure but with a systolic reading of >70 mmHg, malaise without loss of consciousness, anxiety reaction
- Cutaneous or mucosal manifestations: urticaria, angioedema
- Respiratory signs: "asthma-like" dyspnea or difficult breathing related to obstruction of the upper airways, such as edema of the larynx. Sometimes the patient develops a dry, whooping type of cough or bronchial hypersecretion.

Course

The first 30–60 minutes are the most critical. Beyond that time, the condition is usually reversible. However, certain severe forms may necessitate treatment and observation for at least 24 hours.

The most severe forms are generally the ones that have developed most rapidly after exposure to the precipitating factor.

Circumstances of onset

By definition, anaphylactic shock cannot occur with the first administration of a product. Shock

The electrocardiogram may show flattening and inversion of the T wave, ST segment elevation or depression, arrhythmia.

The precipitating factor appears to influence the chances of a fatal outcome.

Any treatment with beta-blockers risks a severe reaction.

following an initial exposure is the result of an idiosyncratic reaction or of possible cross allergies.

The reaction most generally occurs at the beginning of a second or subsequent course of treatment. However, cases occurring in the middle of a treatment have been reported.

The route of administration is important, and shock is more frequent and more severe following an injection. However, a number of drugs administered orally (as well as foods) may precipitate shock.

Evidence implicating a drug

- The most telling evidence is based on the **time of onset**: most anaphylactic shocks occur in a matter of minutes or within the first 2 hours following oral or parenteral administration.
- An inquiry must also be made regarding a past history of sensitization, especially one that has elicited minor signs of allergy.
- Known cases of anaphylactic shock attributed to the same agent constitute a strong argument.
- Other possible causes of shock must be considered:
  - non drug-related anaphylaxis, induced for example by food (strawberries, peanuts) or caused by Hymenoptera stings
  - cardiogenic: myocardial infarction, or arrhythmia, or conduction disorders

  - hypovolemic: the context is generally very suggestive.

The absence of signs of skin or mucosal allergy does not rule out anaphylactic shock.

The emergency setting in which acute cardiocirculatory distress must be managed is not always conducive to the collection of all useful information, particularly ECG data. In addition, anaphylactic shock may produce ECG abnormalities or even ischemic lesions.

Principal causative agents

- Diagnostic products: iodinated radiologic contrast media
- Analgesics and NSAIDs: glafenine and derivatives, aspirin, all NSAIDs and narcotic (opioid) analgesics
- Antibiotics: especially beta-lactams
- Large molecules: blood, serum or derived products, vaccines
- Enzymes.

Also:

- *certain hormones: ACTH, insulin, calcitonin*
- *local anesthetics*
- *various: preservatives and colorants (dyes), neuromuscular blocking drugs, sulfonamides, vitamins B1 and B12, cancer chemotherapy.*

Management

Anaphylactic reactions are often unpredictable. Still, prophylactic measures should not be neglected whenever they can be used. After the offending drug has been identified, the patient should be made aware of the risks of readministration. An entry to that effect should be made in the patient's medical records, listing the different proprietary drugs that contain the active principle responsible. If the medication is indispensable, desensitization may be considered.

The management of anaphylactic shock has to be tailored to the severity of the reaction. The physician does not necessarily carry with him all the requisite supplies, and a call to a well-equipped CPR unit is often the first action to be taken. In the interim, certain life support measures can be applied to maintain tissue perfusion and ventricular ejection: place the patient in a supine position with the legs elevated; most importantly, administer 0.25–1 mg of epinephrine i.v. and restore the intravascular volume. Combined treatment with antihistamines and corticosteroids can be used secondarily to prevent or control certain events such as bronchospasm. It may be advisable to carry out continuing observation for 24 hours because of delayed effects.

References

Bochner BS, Lichtenstein LM. Anaphylaxis. New Engl J Med 1991; 324: 1785–90.

Charpin J. Allergologie. Paris: Flammarion Médecine-Sciences, 1986: 1024.

de Weck AL, Bungaard H. Allergic Reactions to Drugs. Berlin: Springer Verlag, 1983: 752.

5 Acute renal failure

Eugène Rothschild

Definitions

Renal failure (RF) (or renal insufficiency) is defined as a reduction in the glomerular filtration rate.

Acute renal failure (ARF) is a rapid deterioration in renal function, in which the glomerular filtration rate (GFR) decreases within hours or days.

In **intrinsic ARF**, structural lesions are present whose initial localization is the basis for the classification of the variety of nephropathy: tubular, interstitial, vascular or glomerular. **Prerenal failure**, in contrast to intrinsic ARF, is characterized by the absence of histologic renal lesions. Prerenal failure is due to renal hypoperfusion.

Diagnosis

Aside from the existence of **anuria, renal failure is diagnosed through laboratory tests.**

Anuria is defined as the absence of urine output without urinary retention.

It is based on the quantitative determination of **serum creatinine.**

The serum creatinine level depends not only on the GFR but also on the muscle mass, which varies with the individual and according to sex and age.

Thus, the diagnosis of RF can be further delineated by calculating the **creatinine clearance**. In daily practice it can be estimated by nomograms, such as the Cockcroft and Gault formula:

Factor K is equal to 0.814 if the serum creatinine level is expressed in μmol/L, and 7.2 if it is expressed in mg/L; in women, the result has to be multiplied by 0.85.

$$\text{creatinine clearance (ml/min)} = \frac{\text{weight (kg)} \times (140 - \text{age})}{K \times \text{serum creatinine}}$$

Adverse Drug Reactions. A Practical Guide to Diagnosis and Management. Edited by C. Bénichou.
©1994 John Wiley & Sons Ltd.

In certain conditions, the elevation in serum creatinine does not reflect a decrease in the GFR.

The increased serum creatinine value may be an actual rise due to:

- increased creatinine production: rhabdomyolysis, catabolism of nitrogenous compounds (severe febrile illness, extensive burns).
- decreased renal tubular secretion of creatinine: cimetidine, trimethoprim, probenecid.

Interference in colorimetric determination may give a false reading of the creatinine. These chromogens include the following:

- *Endogenous substances:*
  - *acetoacetate (in diabetic ketoacidosis)*
  - *marked hyperglycemia*
  - *marked hyperuricemia*
- *Exogenous compounds:*
  - *certain cephalosporins*

This is where **BUN (blood urea nitrogen)** determination is particularly useful. However, it is less reliable as an index of the GFR because the plasma concentration of urea is also influenced by urine output and nitrogen balance.

*It should be noted, however, that **actual acute renal failure may be present** in some of these circumstances (rhabdomyolysis, diabetic coma, acute tubulointerstitial nephritis caused by some of the drugs previously mentioned).*

Diagnostic criteria

Because of the necessity for unambiguous parameters to define renal failure (RF), relatively high "threshold" values have been proposed; as a result, a certain number of authentic cases may be overlooked.

No definite level of pathological significance can be set for creatinine (or urea). Thus, a serum creatinine level of 130 μmol/L may have no pathological significance in a young man with a large muscle mass, while 90 μmol/L may reflect already appreciable RF in a small elderly woman.

- A diagnosis of **renal failure** can be accepted in three circumstances:
  - Serum creatinine: $\geqslant 150$ μmol/L
  or
  - Creatinine clearance: $\leqslant 50$ mL/min
  or
  - Urea nitrogen $\geqslant 17$ mmol/L

- When the records of repeated test results over time are available, the diagnosis of **acute renal** insufficiency, when stringent criteria are adopted is limited to the two following circumstances:
  - **a rise in serum creatinine** of more than 50% over a previous value determined within the past 6 months,
  or
  - **the presence of renal failure** (as defined above) **plus a rise in urea nitrogen** of more than 100% over a previous value determined within the past 6 months.

However, when the focus is on **diagnostic sensitivity** (especially if other signs of acute renal damage are also present), the diagnosis of acute renal failure can be based on a rise of 30% in serum creatinine (or a decrease of 30% in creatinine clearance) and a rise of 60% in urea nitrogen.

Distinction between intrinsic and prerenal ARF

Differential diagnosis is required mainly when oliguria is present. **Definite evidence of intrinsic ARF is provided by the demonstration of histologic renal lesions.** In clinical practice, unless a renal biopsy is performed, it is often difficult to make a definite distinction between an intrinsic ARF and a prerenal disorder, particularly since the cause is the same in certain cases. The following may be helpful:

- **Clinical data**
  - **context**: a situation in which it is known that a reduction in renal blood flow may be present raises the possibility of prerenal failure

*It is easier to interpret the serum creatinine and urea nitrogen values **when, rather than depending on a single result, a series of determinations over the course of time is available**, especially when the tests were performed shortly before the initiating event. The diagnosis of renal failure may then be established based on levels lower than the ones referred to above, and it can also be determined that the failure is acute.*

Oliguria is present in about 50% of cases of ARF.

Causes of prerenal failure

- *Extracellular dehydration (sodium-free diet, diarrhea, vomiting, extensive burns, etc.)*

Table 1 Indices for differentiating between intrinsic and prerenal acute renal failure

	Intrinsic ARF	Mechanism undetermined	Prerenal ARF
$\dfrac{\text{S urea} \quad \mu\text{mol/L}}{\text{S creat} \quad \mu\text{mol/L}}$	<60	60–80	>80
$\dfrac{U}{S}$ urea	<8	8–10	>10
$\dfrac{U}{S}$ creatinine	<20	20–40	>40
$\dfrac{U}{S}$ osmolar	<1.1	1.1–1.3	>1.3
Urinary osmolality (mOsm/kg)	<350	350–500	>500
UNa (mmol/L)*	>40	20–40	<20
$F_E\text{Na}^* = \dfrac{\text{UNa} \times \text{S creat}}{\text{PNa} \times \text{U creat}} \times 100$	>1	—	<1
$\text{RFI}^* = \dfrac{\text{UNa} \times \text{S creat}}{\text{U creat}}$	>1	—	<1

U = urinary concentration
S = serum concentration
F_ENa = fractional excretion of sodium
RFI = renal failure index
*These indices are interpretable only in patients on a normal sodium diet and who are not on diuretic treatment.

- **signs and symptoms**: the occurrence of the following abnormalities suggests an intrinsic ARF:
  - arterial hypertension
  - proteinuria >1 g/24 hours (aside from cases of acute heart failure)
  - hematuria
- **Laboratory findings**
  The classic criteria are given in Table 1: they are not unfailingly reliable.
- **A test treatment** applied in circumstances that suggest prerenal acute failure. When, after the cause has been eradicated or corrected:
  - a reduction of at least 33% in the serum creatinine level or of at least 50% in BUN occurs within 24 hours, a prerenal type of disorder is confirmed

- *Reduced circulating blood volume (edema, low cardiac output, hemorrhage, vascular sequestration in a context of hypovolemic shock or severe infection)*
- *Hypotension*
- *Renal artery obstruction*

- intrinsic ARF is present when the serum creatinine level continues to rise after 72 hours
- in all other situations, no conclusion can be drawn on the nature of the disorder.

Criteria of severity

Some clinical findings are of **immediate and serious concern**, requiring consultation with a specialist: severe or rapidly progressive RF; anuria; the consequences of RF with circulatory overload (acute arterial hypertension, water and salt retention); fluid and electrolyte disturbances (hyponatremia, hyperkalemia, metabolic acidosis); other organ damage.

*Two **criteria of severity** can be recognized* a posteriori:

- *the necessity for dialysis during the acute episode*
- *the persistence beyond 6 months of renal impairment or the aggravation of pre-existing RF*

Evidence for implicating a drug

Drugs are currently responsible for about 20% of the cases of ARF observed in departments of nephrology; this percentage is even higher if those caused by iodinated radiocontrast media are included. This figure takes into account mainly hospitalized cases. On the other hand, a recent epidemiological study conducted in the USA has shown that drug-induced parenchymal nephropathies involving ambulatory patients free of pre-existing renal disease and requiring hospitalization are unusual in the general population.

Prerenal ARF

Drugs that may induce prerenal failure include agents causing renal hypoperfusion (diuretics, interleukin 2) and also those producing intrarenal hemodynamic changes (angiotensin-converting enzyme inhibitors, NSAIDs, cyclosporin). Their action is pharmacological; there is an increased risk of ARF in those conditions (mentioned above) where renal blood flow is reduced.

The test treatment, in this context, consists of dechallenge, together with volume expansion if need be. In certain cases where continuation of the treatment is considered essential (diuretic treatment, cyclosporin, interleukin 2), a reduction in dosage may suffice.

Intrinsic ARF

In essence, there are two principal types of mechanisms for drug-induced acute renal failure: **direct toxicity** or **hypersensitivity** (other, indirect mechanisms may be involved, such as tubular obstruction, immunohemolytic anemia, rhabdomyolysis).

As far as lesions are concerned, direct toxicity produces acute tubular necrosis or, much more rarely, acute vascular nephropathy; hypersensitivity reactions commonly produce acute tubulointerstitial nephritis, sometimes vasculitis and, exceptionally, isolated acute glomerular nephropathy.

The **clinical features** of the acute nephropathy may provide a clue to the causative mechanism: an isolated ARF, whether or not accompanied by renal shutdown, is usually a manifestation of toxic acute tubular necrosis; the coexistence of marked proteinuria and/or urinary abnormalities (hematuria, leukocyturia, eosinophiluria) and/or hypertension and/or extrarenal signs (fever, arthralgia, rash, eosinophilia, abnormal liver tests) tends to indicate that the nephropathy is caused by hypersensitivity.

However, there is no strict parallel between the anatomic and clinical findings, and, ultimately, the only way to demonstrate the particular histologic variety of nephropathy with certainty is to perform a renal biopsy.

More than 100 drugs have been incriminated in the development of ARF. Antibiotics are implicated in 40–50% of cases of drug-induced ARF. With certain agents, the occurrence of toxic insult is frequent and relatively reproducible, particularly when certain predisposing factors are present (see below). For example, it has been estimated that 15% of patients treated with aminoglycoside antibiotics may develop an aminoglycoside-induced

ARF; this risk rises to 80% for amphotericin B. In contrast, other drugs are very rarely involved: even though some 50 drugs have been incriminated in the occurrence of acute interstitial nephritis (due to individual hypersensitivity), the cases reported have been few, even anecdotal.

Evidence implicating a drug in the occurrence of intrinsic ARF

Two types of data must be sought simultaneously: positive evidence, relating to the drugs involved, and negative evidence that goes to make up the etiologic diagnosis.

Positive evidence

In case of overdosage

Overdosage (deliberate or accidental) with an agent known as a nephrotoxin is useful evidence for the diagnosis of dose-dependent, toxic ARF.

Time to onset

The physician is entitled to suspect that a drug is responsible when ARF occurs **after the start of the treatment** or develops **less than 48 hours after its discontinuation**. In the case of agents with a long half-life, the 48-hour "countdown" begins at the time that the drug is presumed to have been eliminated from the body (in practice, five half-lives).

We should bear in mind that RF may continue to worsen even though treatment has been discontinued (and that only then will serum creatinine exceed the 150 μmol/L threshold) in the case of certain drugs that accumulate in the renal cortex, such as aminoglycosides. With some short, repeated courses of treatment, the detection of renal failure (whether or not it is expressed as an acute disorder) may even be delayed for several months, as with mitomycin C or certain nitrosoureas, for instance.

Clinical pattern

No clinical signs or symptoms are pathognomonic of a drug-related origin for ARF. However, close

The same drug may cause different varieties of acute nephropathy.

associations have been noted between certain drugs and a preferential clinical pattern of ARF.

The association of a nephrotic syndrome with acute interstitial nephritis (which occurs especially in relation to certain NSAIDs) is **highly suggestive of a drug-related origin**.

The following are also **indicative**:

- Concomitant skin rash or liver damage, elevation of serum IgE, eosinophilia, eosinophiluria
- Circulating antibodies to renal tubular basement membranes detected transiently in the context of acute tubulointerstitial nephritis
- Histologically, in the context of acute tubulointerstitial nephritis, the presence in the renal interstitium of epithelial granulomata, eosinophils or IgE-bearing plasma cells, of antibody deposits displaying a linear pattern along the tubular basement membranes under immunofluorescence examination.

There is no test specific for a drug-related origin. This applies in particular to immunologic tests (in vitro lymphocyte stimulation test, inhibition of leukocyte migration, basophil degranulation or histamine release); such positive test results are insufficient grounds for incriminating the drug in the onset of ARF. However, the demonstration of **antibodies directed against a drug** *(or one of its metabolites) and the interaction between these antibodies, red blood cells and the drug (or its metabolite) is valuable evidence for the etiologic diagnosis of ARF associated with immune hemolytic anemia.*

Circumstantial evidence inherent in the patient or the context

These risk factors for ARF (see column opposite) are involved essentially in direct nephrotoxicity. They are particularly well known in connection with aminoglycosides.

Risk factors in aminoglycoside nephrotoxicity

- *Factors related to the patient:*
  - *advanced age*
  - *pre-existing chronic renal failure*
  - *sodium depletion*
  - *liver cirrhosis*
- *Factors related to the context:*
  - *concomitant administration of other potentially nephrotoxic drugs (NSAIDs, diuretics, cyclosporin, certain cephalosporins) or iodinated radiocontrast media*

Table 2 Principal causes of renal failure with acute presentation

Acute tubular necrosis
Shock, infection and all causes of uncorrected prerenal failure
Hemolysis
Rhabdomyolysis
Toxic agents

Acute (tubulo)interstitial nephritis

Infectious diseases	acute pyelonephritis
	systemic infections (bacterial, spirochetal, viral, parasitic)
Immune disorders	systemic lupus erythematosus
	sarcoidosis
	Sjögren's syndrome
Metabolic disorders	hypercalcemia
	acute hyperuricemia
	primary hyperoxaluria
Malignant disorders	lymphoma
	acute leukemia
Idiopathic nephritis	with or without uveitis

Acute glomerulonephritis
Acute post streptococcal glomerulonephritis
Subacute endocarditis
Septicemia, deep-seated sepsis
Systemic lupus erythematosus
Mixed cryoglobulinemia
Goodpasture's syndrome
Crescentic extracapillary glomerulonephritis

Necrotizing vasculitis
Henoch–Schönlein purpura
Polyarteritis nodosa
Wegener vasculitis

Vascular diseases
Malignant hypertension
Scleroderma
Hemolytic-uremic syndrome
Thrombotic thrombocytopenic purpura
Radiation nephritis
Cholesterol emboli syndrome

Myeloma

Obstruction:
Of urinary outflow
Of renal veins
Of renal arteries

- *Factors related to the drug:*
  - *high doses*
  - *prolonged administration*
  - *repeated treatment courses given at close intervals*

Negative evidence

The negative evidence consists of findings pointing to a **non drug-related cause**. Theoretically, a drug-related explanation can only be confirmed after the other possible causes of ARF (which are statistically more frequent than the drug-induced causes) have been eliminated. Table 2 shows the other principal diagnoses to be considered in renal failure with an acute onset.

The very diversity of the causes of ARF accounts for the fact that it is frequently difficult or impossible to obtain immediate exhaustive information to either rule in or rule out the implication of drugs. However, there are certain data that constitute the **minimum information** always necessary to assess the role of a drug and identify an intrinsic renal disorder (i.e. excluding prerenal factors and urinary obstruction).

Minimum information required:

- *state of hydration: blood pressure, body weight, laboratory parameters (serum sodium, protein or albumin, hematocrit or hemoglobin level), examination of the skin, and any changes in these findings*
- *data on known infection and fever, cardiocirculatory status (recent history of circulatory failure, heart failure)*
- *rule out urinary tract obstruction (by renal ultrasound examination).*

Practical considerations

Sometimes, drug involvement appears highly probable:

- When an intentional or accidental **overdosage** of a **known nephrotoxin** appears obvious. Sometimes, an overdosage can be confirmed only by determining the drug concentration in the serum.

- When a **recurrence** of ARF occurs with the **reintroduction** of the same

However, bear in mind that an excessive serum level of the suspect drug may simply be due to its accumulation resulting from renal failure whose cause is quite different.

drug, in the same circumstances. In this case, a time of onset of less than 4 days is suggestive.

Obviously, in these cases, it is **imperative that the suspect drug be discontinued**, and, if a **hypersensitivity reaction** is involved, that it be **withdrawn permanently.**

The drug's role can be reasonably ruled out

- If the drug treatment **began after** the onset of ARF or was discontinued **more than 48 hours** before.
- If **another cause of ARF** is demonstrated rapidly. In these cases, it is permissible to continue or to reintroduce the drug treatment.
- **Improvement in renal function** while the drug is continued at the same dose rules out the possibility of drug-induced **intrinsic ARF.**

In other cases

The involvement of the drug cannot be excluded or confirmed. The causality assessment is a matter of probability: the role of the drug is suggested on the basis of the time sequence and suspicion will be stronger or weaker according to the evidence provided by the situation and by what is known concerning the agent's toxicity. In practice:

It is preferable as a matter of principle to discontinue any drug that is not vitally necessary, while refraining from improperly withdrawing a drug that might be the only possible treatment for the cause of the ARF.

Thus, for example, the development of RF during a treatment for severe infection might be due to the antibiotics or to an undetected focus of infection persisting as a result of inadequate or inappropriate treatment. In a patient with heart failure, the onset of RF while on diuretics might reflect excessive sodium depletion but could also be caused by a hemodynamic deterioration that would not justify the suspension of diuretics.

Early withdrawal of the offending drug is usually the best way to guarantee total recovery without sequelae and is often the only therapeutic measure required.

Particularly when it is necessary to continue the treatment (or when its reintroduction at a later time is contemplated), it is important to try to determine whether the adverse reaction's mechanism is common to the therapeutic class or pharmacological family to which the causative agent belongs. This may involve the pharmacodynamic mode of action (for example, ARF caused by any of the angiotensin-converting enzyme inhibitors in the event of bilateral renal artery stenosis), or possibly cross-allergy. On the contrary, it could be a hypersensitivity reaction to a particular agent. In the former case, no drug belonging to the same family may be substituted; in the latter case, if the immunogenic part of the molecule of the medication is known, it may sometimes be possible to replace it by a related drug (for example, in certain cases of acute tubulointerstitial nephritis caused by rifampicin, it has been possible to continue the antitubercular treatment uneventfully with rifamycin SV).

In all cases, the course must be followed.

Spontaneous recovery of renal function on discontinuation of the treatment lends support to a relationship with the drug: thus, the course is **suggestive of a drug-related causation** *a posteriori* if renal function improves within ten days of discontinuation of the drug (or a reduction in its dosage).

Conversely, a diagnosis may sometimes be corrected and reversed a posteriori when certain laboratory results are eventually obtained (e.g. serum complement determination, tests for autoantibodies, immunoelectrophoresis).

References

Beard K, Perera DR, Jick H. Drug-induced parenchymal renal disease in outpatients. J Clin Pharmacol 1988; 28: 431–5.

Bennett WM, Elzinga LW, Porter GA. Tubulointerstitial disease and toxic nephropathy. In: Brenner BM, Rector FC Jr, eds. The Kidney. Philadelphia: WB Saunders Company, 1991: 1430–96.

Brochner-Mortensen J. Routine methods and their reliability for assessment of glomerular filtration rate in adults. Dan Med Bull 1978; 25: 181–202.

Degaichia A, Vonlanthen M, Agrafiotis A, Rottembourg J, Degoulet P, Jacobs C. Insuffissances rénales aiguës de cause médicale. Aspects cliniques et thérapeutiques chez 142 malades traités dans un service de néphrologie. In: Kuss R, Legrain M, eds. Séminaires d'uro-néphrologie. Paris: Masson, 1981: 187–201.

Hoitsma AJ, Wetzels JFM, Koene RAP. Drug-induced nephrotoxicity. Aetiology, clinical features and management. Drug Safety 1991; 6: 131–47.

Kleinknecht D, Landais P, Goldfarb B. Les insuffissances rénales aiguës associées à des médicaments ou à des produits de contraste iodés. Résultats d'une enquête coopérative multicentrique de la Société de Néphrologie. Néphrologie 1986; 7: 41–6.

Vigeral P, Baumelou A, Bénichou C, Castot A, Danan G, Kreft-Jais C, Lagier G, Rothschild E, Druet P, Grünfeld JP. Les insuffisances rénales d'origine médicamenteuse. Résultats de réunions de consensus. Néphrologie 1989; 10: 157–61.

RENAL FUNCTION ABNORMALITIES

Renal failure

A given blood creatinine (or urea nitrogen) concentration is not indicative of the same renal function level from one patient to the next. Thus, there is no clear, absolute way to define the upper limit of normal for these two parameters. With the aim not to overdiagnose renal failure, relatively high "threshold" values have to be set.

A diagnosis of **renal failure** can be made when the laboratory values indicate:

- serum creatinine $\geqslant 150$ μmol/L

- or serum urea $\geqslant 17$ mmol/L

- or creatinine clearance $\leqslant 50$ ml/min

For other abnormalities, use the following terms:

Serum creatinine increased

Rise in serum creatinine: but the increase remains below 150 μmol/L

Urea serum increased

Rise in serum urea: but the increase remains below 17 mmol/L

Only histologic evidence obtained by renal biopsy can delineate the exact nature of a nephropathy

ACUTE RENAL FAILURE
CHRONOLOGICAL CRITERIA

		Very suggestive	Suggestive	Compatible	Inconclusive	Incompatible
Time to onset of the reaction	Initial treatment or subsequent treatment without previous history			*From start of drug administration* All time intervals		*With regard to start of drug administration* Drug taken after the onset of the reaction	*From end of drug administration** >2 days
	Subsequent treatment with previous history of acute renal failure in relation to the same drug		*From start of drug administration* ≤4 days	*From start of drug administration* >4 days	*From end of drug administration** ≤2 days	

*Or from the time at which the drug is supposed to have been cleared from the body.

		Very suggestive	Suggestive	Compatible	Inconclusive	Not suggestive
Course of the reaction	Without stopping the drug (unchanged dosage)				No change or Aggravation	Improvement of renal function
	After stopping the drug or decrease of dose		Improvement of renal function withing 10 days*		No change or Aggravation	

*The delay may be longer for drugs that accumulate in the renal cortex, such as aminoglycosides, especially in the elderly.

6 Gastrointestinal disorders

Alex Pariente and Gaby Danan

Dysphagia and esophageal symptoms

Definitions

Dysphagia is a sensation of difficulty in swallowing.

Odynophagia is painful swallowing.

Pyrosis (heartburn) is a burning, radiating discomfort arising in the retrosternal region.

Regurgitation is a return of solid or liquid gastric contents into the mouth without the forceful expulsion of vomiting.

Causes
The principal non drug-related causes of dysphagia are:

- *tumors, and especially cancer when dysphagia is **painless** and **progressive,** first involving solids and ultimately liquids.*
- *reflux esophagitis may be progressive and painless, without a **clear-cut history of severe reflux** (one case out of two); or it may follow or **be accompanied by symptoms of reflux** (heartburn, regurgitation) and **odynophagia**;*
- *motor disorders: achalasia, spasms at different levels, "nutcracker" esophagus, are uncommon. Motor dysphagia is often **capricious** and **painful**.*

Drug-induced dysphagia is usually linked to esophageal ulcer.

Drug-induced esophageal ulcer

Ulcer should be suspected immediately on history-taking when **dysphagia appears abruptly after the ingestion of**

Adverse Drug Reactions. A Practical Guide to Diagnosis and Management. Edited by C. Bénichou.
©1994 John Wiley & Sons Ltd.

medications taken without or with very little water, especially at bedtime.

The clinical examination is normal. When **fever or retrosternal chest pain is present, perforation (an exceptional event)** should be suspected and the patient should be hospitalized immediately.

In the case of a severe pain in the anterior thoracic region ruling out a cardiovascular cause (myocardial infarction in particular) is necessary.

Time to onset

A few minutes or hours after ingesting the drug.

Diagnosis

The diagnosis is confirmed by **endoscopy,** which reveals one or more superficial ulcerations at the level of the aortic arch and sometimes above the cardia.

*A subsequent **esophageal stricture** may be the first lesion to be disclosed when the initial episode has gone undetected.*

Causative medicines

Capsules have been incriminated more often than other dosage forms. More than 30 drugs have been implicated.

Treatment

This consists of discontinuing the offending drug, prescription of a liquid or mixed diet, administration of lidocaine jelly (or viscous solution) for pain.

The drug need not be contraindicated subsequently provided that these preventive measures are observed.

As **prevention**, patients should always take two glasses of water and avoid immediate recumbency after taking a medication by mouth.

Other causes of drug-induced dysphagia

Candida (monilial) esophagitis associated with drug treatment

These can appear as dysphagia, odynophagia, or remain latent.

Oral thrush may or may not be present.

At present, the most effective treatment is fluconazole, to be administered for 5 days or more in immunocompromised patients.

Treatments that favor candidiasis include antibiotics, corticosteroids and immunosuppressive drugs.

Other mechanisms

A number of drugs have the potential to **alter esophageal motility** and **promote reflux**: e.g. calcium channel blockers, anticholinergics.

It is possible, though yet unproved, that **aspirin** and **NSAIDs** may aggravate the symptoms or complications of reflux esophagitis.

Esophageal obstruction has been observed after ingestion of dietary fiber and bulk-forming laxatives, especially in elderly individuals or patients with esophageal stricture or motor disorders.

Reference

Weinbeck M, Berges W, Lübke HJ. Drug-induced oesophageal lesions. Baillière's Clin Gastroenterol 1988; 2: 263–74.

Epigastric pain

The main causes of epigastric pain are peptic ulcer, gastroesophageal reflux, gallstones, certain diseases of the liver, pancreatic disorders, diseases of the colon, coronary insufficiency or, fairly frequently, functional disorders. Here, only gastroduodenal, biliary and pancreatic disorders will be discussed.

When analyzing epigastric pain, the radiation of pain, duration, periodicity, precipitating factors, any factor relieving the pain, and associated symptoms need to be considered.

Gastroduodenal lesions

Epigastric pain is a common symptom—sometimes transient—associated with the absorption of almost all drugs and even placebo. In practice, the problem is connected mostly with lesions induced by nonsteroidal anti-inflammatory drugs (NSAIDs), including aspirin.

IMPORTANT:
__Perforations__ can be easily missed on abdominal examination: do not hesitate to order a plain film of the abdomen.

__Bleeding__, occurring as melena, is often missed, especially in elderly patients; it is easily recognized by digital rectal examination.

Aspirin and NSAIDs are responsible for the occurrence of gastroduodenal lesions ranging from erythema to ulceration or the aggravation of a pre-existing peptic ulcer.

In contrast, corticosteroids can be responsible for gastroduodenal lesions only at high doses and/or when cumulative doses are raised.

Management

If the symptoms are mild and of brief duration in a healthy individual with no history of ulcer and whose treatment can be discontinued immediately, it is reasonable to prescribe a simple antacid, sucralfate or even an H_2-receptor antagonist for a short time.

If the symptoms are severe, prolonged, or occur in a patient with a past history of ulcer:

- *__Upper gastrointestinal endoscopy__ is necessary to confirm the presence of lesions, determine their type, number and severity, and rule out other diseases (such as cancer).*

— *if there is no ulceration,* a simple symptomatic treatment may be prescribed;

— if an *ulcerative lesion* is found, the treatment is the same as for a common ulcer. NSAIDs must be withdrawn except when their use is practically mandatory (e.g. in rheumatoid arthritis); their continued administration does not however appear to interfere markedly with healing while the patient is on sucralfate, an H_2-receptor antagonist or a proton pump inhibitor.

Prevention

NSAIDs should be avoided:

- if the patient has a history of ulcer
- in patients over 70 years of age
- as unsupervised long-term treatment.

The patients should be advised to watch for warning signs: epigastric pain, melena.

The only drug recognized to prevent lesions induced by NSAIDs is misoprostol at a dose of 200 µg 2–4 times daily. However, this treatment may cause diarrhea and pain and should be **reserved for long-term treatments and elderly patients**.

Reference

The NSAIDs and the Gastrointestinal Mucosa. Scand J Gastroenterol 1988; 24 (suppl 163): 1–72.

Biliary and pancreatic pain

The clinical features are immediately suggestive and call for a plain film of the abdomen, an ultrasound examination, a serum amylase or lipase determination and a hepatic work-up.

Gallstone formation is promoted by plasma cholesterol lowering agents (except HMG-CoA reductase inhibitors), by estrogens and by cholestyramine. Very small stones may be hard to detect by ultrasound but can easily create problems as they pass from the gallbladder or can cause pancreatitis. It is reasonable to perform an ultrasound examination before undertaking treatment with these drugs.

Certain drugs or their metabolites can precipitate or promote precipitation of certain substances in the bile and produce an image of sludge on the ultrasonogram. This is usually reversible on discontinuation of the treatment.

Acute pancreatitis can be produced by drugs. After eliminating the usual causes (alcoholism, cholelithiasis) or the less common ones (trauma, hypertriglyceridemia, hypercalcemia, viral pancreatitis), a possible association with medicines taken should be suspected after assessing the timing and information from specialists and/or data banks.

Reference

Mallory A, Kern F. Drug-induced pancreatitis. Baillière's Clin Gastroenterol 1988; 2: 293–308.

Constipation

Definition

There is no satisfactory general definition of constipation. The essential feature is **decreased motility**: stools are less frequent, harder and/or more difficult to void.

Constipation is frequently associated with other symptoms: pain, bloating and even nausea.

It may be severe and eventually result in actual functional obstruction.

Causative agents

Drugs whose action directly affects luminal fecal content: e.g. aluminum hydroxide, sucralfate, cholestyramine.

Drugs that act on the autonomic nervous system, such as clonidine, opiates, anticholinergics (antimuscarinic agents), tricyclic antidepressants, antipsychotics.

Management

In the event of severe abdominal distension and/or vomiting, the patient should be hospitalized.

When a drug treatment cannot be suspended or substituted (e.g. long-term antipsychotic therapy), the constipation must be treated: abundant fluids, dietary fiber, osmotic laxatives and rectal medications if necessary.

Whenever possible, discontinuation of the suspect drug is desirable.

Rectal examination is mandatory so that a fecaloma will not be overlooked.

One should be alert for an organic cause that may be associated with constipation, particularly with a disorder of recent onset occurring in the course of long-term treatment. In addition to the clinical examination, a more detailed evaluation, including a colonoscopy would be reasonable in patients of more than 45 years of age.

Reference

Ewe K. Diarrhoea and constipation. Baillière's Clin Gastroenterol 1988; 2: 353–84.

Diarrhea and pseudomembranous colitis

Definition

Diarrhea is defined as the discharge of more than six soft stools in 36 hours.

*In practice, the important information pertains to a **change** in the frequency of bowel movements and/or the consistency of stools in relation to the previous pattern.*

Signs of severity

- Dehydration and collapse
- Rectal bleeding (hematochezia)
- Fever for more than 48 hours
- Abdominal distension and diminished bowel sounds can signify acute colonic distension.

In the presence of any of these signs, the patient should be hospitalized.

Diarrhea on antibiotics

This should systematically suggest **pseudomembranous colitis (PMC)** caused by the selection of a toxin-secreting anaerobic bacillus, *Clostridium difficile*.

Diarrhea without signs of severity persisting for at least 48 hours justifies discontinuing the antibiotic, which will bring about a resolution in most cases.

Diagnosis of PMC

The onset of diarrhea may occur during treatment, early but also **after the end** of antibiotic therapy (up to 3 weeks later).

PMC may also be observed after treatment with anticancer drugs, in association with diseases that produce segmental narrowing of the colon, or spontaneously, sometimes in epidemic fashion.

The onset is abrupt, with the discharge of large numbers of liquid stools, often accompanied by colic. Fever is present in one case out of four.

The clinical manifestations can range from the absence of diarrhea to severe PMC, complicated by toxic megacolon and even perforation of the colon.

Colonoscopy reveals characteristic pseudomembranes; the rectum and the sigmoid colon are involved in 90% of cases.

Colonoscopy can also rule out other causes of colitis: infection, ischemia, inflammatory bowel diseases or tumor.

Management

Antibiotic treatment must be suspended immediately.

Drugs that decrease gastrointestinal motility (muscarinic blocking agents, narcotic analgesics, antidiarrheal drugs) **must not be given**.

They increase the risk of colon distention and the time of contact with the toxin.

For treatment, use **oral vancomycin** at a dose of 125–500 mg four times daily for 7 days, or metronidazole (500 mg three times daily for 7 days).

Recurrences are possible after the treatment is stopped and will usually necessitate more complex treatment regimens.

Prophylactic measures

Hygienic measures for those close to the patient:

- washing of hands
- disinfection of soiled linen and material.

This is particularly important in institutions and other closely associated groups of people.

Hemorrhagic colitis

These cases are more uncommon and are mainly observed with certain penicillins.

They are not caused by Clostridium difficile.

Blood-tinged diarrheal stools appear during the first days of the treatment, with strong colicky pains.

Colonoscopy shows a diffusely edematous, purpuric and congestive appearance, frequently predominating in the right colon. Klebsiella oxytoca is frequently isolated from stools.

Withdrawal of the antibiotic is sufficient to bring about a rapid resolution of the symptoms.

Diarrhea not associated with antibiotics

All types of diarrhea may be caused by drugs.

Generally, there are no macroscopic intestinal lesions. However, ulcerations may occur, for example with NSAIDs, potassium, gold salts.

The temporal relationship between the start of the treatment and the diarrhea is usually obvious.

The diarrhea subsides rapidly after the drug is discontinued, which will obviate the need for investigations into the mechanism of the diarrhea, if the drug-related cause is not recognized immediately.

References

Ewe K. Diarrhoea and constipation. Baillière's Clin Gastroenterol 1988; 2: 353–84.

Lembcke B, Caspary WF. Malabsorption syndromes. Baillière's Clin Gastroenterol 1988; 2: 329–51.

Levecq H, Cerf M. Diarrhée des antibiotiques. Ann Gastroenterol Hepatol 1990; 26: 147–56.

Pariente EA. Entéropathies médicamenteuses. Gastroenterol Clin Biol 1982; 6: 16–18.

7 Respiratory disorders

Michel Fournier

Acute dyspnea

Definition

Acute dyspnea refers to the rapid development of severe respiratory discomfort.

The clinical picture includes:

- **Constant** signs: abnormal resting ventilation, either rapid (polypnea) or slow (inspiratory bradypnea)
- **Variable** signs according to the dyspnea's mechanism.

There are essentially two kinds of mechanism of drug-related acute dyspnea:

- *an **obstruction** to airflow in the conducting portion of the respiratory tract; it may be localized (laryngeal edema) or diffuse (asthma attack);*
- ***deterioration in gas exchange**, such as those observed in diffuse interstitial lung disorders.*

Dyspnea is not always linked to respiratory insufficiency

Drugs may impair ventilation and cause alveolar hypoventilation (hypercapnia and hypoxia) without producing a sensation of dyspnea.

They act in the following manner:

- *by depressing the central control of ventilation, with consequences that occur earlier and are more serious in patients with pre-existing respiratory insufficiency (e.g. opiates, hypnotics)*
- *by affecting the neuromuscular junction of respiratory muscles: skeletal muscle relaxants, antibiotics in myasthenia gravis.*

Adverse Drug Reactions. A Practical Guide to Diagnosis and Management. Edited by C. Bénichou.
©1994 John Wiley & Sons Ltd.

Circumstances of diagnosis

Diagnosis of a drug-related cause of
acute dyspnea is not relevant in typical
forms of pulmonary embolism,
myocardial infarction, or hypovolemia
secondary to internal bleeding.

It is principally in atypical forms of the
above-mentioned diseases or with the
onset of acute dyspneic symptoms in a
patient with a dyspnea-producing
cardiac disease that a drug-related
etiology is considered. In such cases, the
most compelling evidence is the
temporal relationship of the events.

Acute dyspnea caused by an obstruction in airflow

Noisy respiration and certain unusual ventilatory characteristics are helpful in:

- Linking the dyspnea to an obstruction in airflow
- Differentiating between laryngotracheal obstructions and bronchial asthma:

	Laryngotracheal obstructions	Asthma
Localization	Larynx, extrathoracic trachea	Intrathoracic airways
Mechanisms of obstruction	Edema, abscess, neoplasms, foreign bodies	Edema, smooth muscle contraction, varying degrees of associated hypersecretion
General symptoms	1. Inspiratory bradypnea 2. In some cases, cough, change in the quality of the voice, pain	1. Polypnea with slowed expiration 2. Cough, expectoration 3. No pain, no change in the quality of the voice

Acute dyspnea of laryngeal origin

A drug-induced etiology is rare but should not be overlooked. It should come to mind
when edema of the laryngeal mucous membranes develops suddenly, namely with the onset
of bradypnea characterized by difficult, prolonged inspiration, associated with:

- more or less extensive edema of the face and neck
- a timing consistent with the administration or reintroduction of a drug
- an atopic background.

This calls for the immediate administration of corticosteroids, plus the injection of epinephrine in case of shock, permanent withdrawal of the causative drug and hospitalization.

The approach to the differential diagnosis differs in adults and in children.

- In children: the causes of acute laryngeal dyspnea unrelated to injury are limited to laryngitis and foreign bodies. Inflammation of the larynx is principally of the following types:

  - subglottic laryngitis of gradual onset in a context of febrile nasopharyngitis

  - laryngitis with stridor, whose onset is more abrupt
  - *Hemophilus influenzae* epiglottitis, with high fever.

- **In adults**: pharyngeal and laryngeal tumors are more common than neurologic causes (amyotrophic lateral sclerosis).

In laryngitis, besides treatment for the infection, corticosteroid therapy is required; it is dangerous to place the child in a supine position.

A laryngeal foreign body has to be considered in a case of acute dyspnea immediately complicating a syndrome de pénétration; in case of extreme emergency, a Heimlich maneuvre should be tried.

Acute dyspnea of bronchial origin

The symptoms are similar to those of an asthma attack: noisy respiration with coarse crackles and wheezes audible to the patient are heard in both lung fields and are intensified during expiration; cough is less prominent, with minimal and difficult expectoration in the latter part of the episode. Cyanosis is limited or absent.

These symptoms of paroxysmal bronchial obstruction are generally easy to distinguish from acute laryngeal dyspnea where the lung bases are clear on auscultation. Auscultation of the upper chest is more problematic because of the production of laryngotracheal sounds; in any event, in asthma, the main respiratory difficulty is on expiration.

The diagnosis of an asthma attack is further facilitated by:

- a history of past attacks, whose pattern is recognized by the patient
- the efficacy of the inhalation of a beta$_2$-adrenergic agent, which reduces the dyspnea within minutes (while this measure is ineffective in laryngeal dyspnea).

The number of causative drugs is small

- Intolerance or allergy to **vehicles for solutions or suspensions of drugs given by inhalation** is easy to recognize; true sensitization is rare; clinically, the precipitation of coughing fits by the inhalation is much more common than the onset of an asthma attack.

- **Intolerance or allergy to the inhaled drugs themselves** manifested as asthma attacks is exceptional (sodium cromoglycate) and requires discontinuation of the treatment.

  The onset of an asthma attack may pose complex problems, since some of these agents (sodium cromoglycate, beta$_2$-adrenergic agents in particular) are supposed to prevent or treat asthma. Changing the drug (and vehicle) generally solves the problem.

- **Converting enzyme inhibitors** may precipitate asthma attacks: this is probably an exceptional situation, and a point of diagnostic significance is that these attacks appear to occur characteristically with the **gradual prior onset of an isolated, dry, chronic cough**.

  *This isolated, dry, chronic cough is a well-known adverse reaction of this class of drugs; it occurs in 5–10% of cases and abates completely and rapidly on discontinuation of the drug. If **absolutely** required by the clinical conditions, another drug of the same therapeutic class can be reintroduced under strict supervision; this measure should be exceptional. This adverse effect is presumed to be caused by an alteration of kinin metabolism.*

Beta-blockers are probably the drugs most often involved in induced asthma: all dosage forms have been implicated (ophthalmic preparations, tablets, injectable solutions).

The mechanism is directly related to the blocking of beta$_2$ receptors of bronchial smooth muscle cells: the effect is therefore reversible as soon as the drug is stopped. This untoward effect of beta-blockers is observed essentially in asthmatics; their use is therefore inadvisable in these patients.

- **NSAIDs, including aspirin,** may trigger attacks of asthma; they occur in predisposed individuals,

  Inhibition of cyclo-oxygenase synthesis is probably not the only mechanism involved.

characterized in the typical forms by nasal polyps and an atopic background; the asthma that is precipitated (and often reactivated) in this way is difficult to control.

Conclusion

Acute drug-induced asthma probably does not occur unpredictably: a known atopic background, even if remote, and of course past episodes of asthma in the patient's history, demand that caution be exercised when prescribing the drugs mentioned above.

It should also be pointed out that the induction mechanisms are not unequivocal or necessarily supported by solid evidence: IgE-dependent sensitization, blocking of beta$_2$ muscle receptors, alteration of prostaglandin or kinin system metabolism.

Acute dyspnea caused by interstitial lung disease

Clinical features

Diagnosis is practically impossible without a chest x-ray, the only helpful sign being diffuse, symmetric or asymmetric crepitant or subcrepitant crackles audible in the lung fields. The breathing is generally rapid, superficial, **without** expiratory slowing, and some degree of cyanosis is usually present.

Radiology

Filled alveoli are superimposed upon an increased reticular pattern and sometimes a micronodular pattern: the complete picture constitutes an alveolar interstitial syndrome.

Analysis of blood gases

Hypoxia and hypocapnia are a usual finding and reflect a sometimes severe shunt effect.

Pulmonary function tests

If the condition of the patient allows pulmonary function tests to be performed, the studies show a decrease in lung volumes (in which FEV_1, VC and TLC are reduced to the same degree), and diffuse interstitial abnormalities (reduction of D_{LCO}).

Etiologic diagnosis

In the clinical picture described, there is nothing that suggests a particular etiology. It is not preceded by nasopharyngitis with fever, there is no known contact pointing to an infectious origin. Furthermore, there is no heart disease, pericarditis (on auscultation, ECG or ultrasound examination) or cardiomegaly. Finally, a knowledge of the few drugs responsible for these acute presentations may lead to the diagnosis: methotrexate, gold salts, nitrofurantoin, sulfonamides, nilutamide.

- It is imperative that the treatment be permanently discontinued, since the outcome may otherwise be fatal.

- High-dose corticosteroid therapy is consistently effective; it is preferable that it be given in a hospital setting.

- In most cases, there are no lasting clinical or radiologic sequelae.

References

Akoun GA, White JP. Treatment-induced Respiratory Disorders. Amsterdam: Elsevier, 1989.

Cooper JAD Jr, White DA, Matthay RA. Drug-induced pulmonary disease. Part 1: Cytotoxic drugs. Am Rev Respir Dis 1986; 133: 321–40. Part 2: Non-cytotoxic drugs. Am Rev Respir Dis 1986; 133: 488–505.

Goldstein RA, Patterson R. Drug allergy: prevention, diagnosis, treatment. J Allergy Clin Immunol Oct 1984; 74 (suppl): 4.

INTERSTITIAL LUNG DISEASE
DEFINITION

The diagnosis of **interstitial lung disease** is:

- **possible** when there are isolated radiologic signs
- **probable** when, in addition to the radiologic abnormalities, the findings include one of the clinical symptoms and one of the functional disorders.

1) *Radiologic signs*

    Type of picture:
- micronodular infiltrative lesions
- and/or reticular infiltrative lesions
- and/or irregular scattered opacities

These may be disseminated, at the onset or progressively.

2) *Clinical symptoms*

    Onset or aggravation of dyspnea and/or cough.

3) *Functional disorders*

- restrictive ventilatory disorder
- and/or reduction of carbon monoxide diffusion of more than 30% in the absence of an obstructive ventilatory disorder
- and/or hypoxia with normocapnia or hypocapnia.

INTERSTITIAL LUNG DISEASE
CHRONOLOGICAL CRITERIA

		Very suggestive	Suggestive	Compatible	Inconclusive	Incompatible
Time to onset of the reaction	Initial treatment			*From start of drug administration* All time intervals		*With regard to start of drug administration* Drug taken after the onset of the reaction
	Subsequent treatment without previous history					
	Subsequent treatment with previous history in relation to the same drug	*From start of drug administration* ⩽2 days		*From start of drug administration* >2 days		

		Very suggestive	Suggestive	Compatible	Inconclusive	Not suggestive
Course of the reaction	Without stopping the drug				Improvement or No change or Aggravation	Durable subsidence within 2 days (with nonsteroidal symptomatic treatment such as diuretics, antibiotics)
	After stopping the drug or decrease of dose		Subsidence of the changes without symptomatic treatment ⩽3 months		Improvement with symptomatic treatment or Improvement >3 months or No improvement	

Drug-induced pleurisy

Diagnostic findings

There are no known specific clinical, biochemical or histologic criteria for linking pleural effusion to the action of a drug. The findings generally include:

- effusion consisting of a small amount of fluid
  - nonproductive cough with lower thoracic pain
  - limited systemic signs, such as moderate fever
  - and association of the effusion with a diffuse interstitial lung disorder.

But the etiologic diagnosis is guided by:

- *negative results of the usual etiologic investigations (sterile effusion, absence of neoplastic pleural cells) and, where indicated, of histologic pleural lesions specific to granuloma formation (either infective, as in tuberculosis, or, uncommonly, referable to sarcoidosis), or else specific to cancer*
- ***and, especially, the temporal relationship to the administration of a drug.***

Two important clinical pictures

Pleuropericarditis of drug-induced lupus erythematosus

The best-known examples are procainamide- and hydralazine-induced lupus.

These cases commonly affect middle-aged individuals and demonstrate symmetric polyarthritis, systemic signs, and **pleuropericarditis**.

All the serologic markers of lupus erythematosus may be present except for hypocomplementemia and anti-DNA and anti-Sm antibodies.

The course is benign and the effusions subside rapidly after the treatment is stopped.

The pleural effusion is moderate and is secondary to the pericarditis.

Pleuritis associated with interstitial lung disorder

It may be an actual diffuse interstitial lung disease or a distention of the interlobular septa appearing on x-ray as Kerley B lines.

When the onset is rapid (after the drug has been taken for a few days), the radiologic and clinical signs abate just as rapidly after administration is discontinued.

Only a small number of cases have been reported. The following agents have been implicated:

- nitrofurantoin and chemically related drugs (dantrolene)
- certain anticancer drugs
- amiodarone, methysergide and bromocriptine.

The volume of the effusion is moderate; either side may be involved.

8 Abnormal blood glucose values

Georges Tchobroutsky

Hypoglycemia

Certain drugs may induce or potentiate hypoglycemia. The diagnostic signs differ depending on whether or not they involve a patient being treated for diabetes mellitus with insulin or with sulfonylureas.

Definition

A distinction is made between hypoglycemia that is preferentially expressed as a result of (carbohydrate) fasting, i.e. at the end of the night, a long time from a meal, aggravated by physical exercise and/or the ingestion of alcohol, and postprandial (reactive) hypoglycemia that occurs after the ingestion of carbohydrates, 2–4 hours after a meal. The latter is very rare, and is diagnosed by the association, during an oral glucose tolerance test, of a low blood glucose level and the symptoms that brought the patient to the physician.

In contrast, in hypoglycemia expressed preferentially in response to fasting—and this is the case of that induced by drugs—the demonstration of a low blood glucose level is sufficient by itself to establish the diagnosis.

Thus, the definition of hypoglycemia is biochemical. The clinical symptomatology may be suggestive, with "malaise", neurologic, mental or psychiatric manifestations without prodromes or sequelae, loss of consciousness and coma, but it is never specific. It cannot therefore be a substitute for laboratory tests. However, it is difficult to set a threshold value for fasting blood glucose that definitely demonstrates its causal relationship with the clinical signs: if below 30 mg/dL, the diagnosis of pathological hypoglycemia is definite; below 50 mg/dL, the diagnosis is only probable; below 60 mg per dL of plasma, determined with glucose oxidase on a venous blood sample, the role of the fall in plasma glucose in causing relevant symptoms merits consideration.

The lower the glucose level and more sensitive to fasting the patient is, the greater the potential risk of coma will be.

Adverse Drug Reactions. A Practical Guide to Diagnosis and Management. Edited by C. Bénichou.
©1994 John Wiley & Sons Ltd.

In patients not treated for diabetes mellitus with insulin or sulfonylureas

All of the hypoglycemic effects, including coma, can be induced by drugs. Drugs occupy a special place in the etiologic investigation. Drugs, alcohol, primary or secondary adrenal insufficiency, a mesenchymal tumor (usually retroperitoneal, intrathoracic or intra-abdominal) must be ruled out systematically before a diagnosis of insulin-secreting pancreatic islet-cell tumor can ultimately be made.

Evidence implicating a drug

The principal presumptive evidence is the sequence of events: namely, the disappearance of hypoglycemia and its effects on withdrawal of the suspect drugs.

The situation is completely different depending on whether the offenders are antidiabetic agents or not.

Antidiabetic agents

In nondiabetics, self-medication with sulfonylureas or insulin is not rare: this may be accidental intoxication, for example by the elderly spouse of a treated diabetic. More often, this is intentional intoxication in a health care professional (pharmacist, physician, nurse, laboratory technician, etc.), in a member of their family or of the family of a treated diabetic. An extreme case of factitious disease is the Münchhausen syndrome (repetitive simulation of serious illness leading to surgical procedures). The strongest evidence of the probability of factitious hypoglycemia is the socio-professional and psychiatric context, negative findings for other causes and, in certain cases where all investigations have culminated in failure, the disappearance of hypoglycemia after strict isolation, e.g. following a 3-day fast in a room alone, without personal belongings.

Insulin self-medication, in a patient who claims that he has never received it, may be detected by the presence of circulating antibodies to insulin. However, these antibodies appear only after weeks of injection and their levels may be undetectable by the usual methods if the insulin is highly purified and has a primary human structure, which is becoming the rule. Another test is to assay plasma collected at presentation of hypoglycemia and look for a high or very high level of circulating insulin with suppressed, undetectable values of C-peptide, an indicator of endogenous insulin secretion.

With sulfonylureas, the test consists of detecting the drug in the urine or blood, when technically feasible.

Other drugs

The situation is completely different: there is no particular psychological or psychiatric profile. Generally, the patients involved are neither health professionals, nor diabetics nor relatives of diabetics. The nature of the offending drugs depends on the disease being treated.

The drugs most often implicated are as follows:

- **In treated diabetics**
  - insulin
  - sulfonylureas
  - agents that potentiate sulfonylureas

- **In all patients (diabetics and nondiabetics)**
  - insulin (taken secretively/injection forgotten?)
  - sulfonylureas (taken secretively or by mistake)
  - salicylates
  - perhexilline
  - propoxyphene
  - disopyramide
  - pentamidine
  - certain MAOIs
  - oxytetracyclines
  - quinine i.v. (and/or acute malaria)
  - certain antithyroid drugs, pyritinol (molecules containing thiol groups)

Molecules containing **thiol groups** are a rare cause in Western Europe but a common one in Japan. These molecules induce anti-insulin antibodies in the absence of a prior injection of insulin. These anti-insulin antibodies are insulin-secreting and therefore hypoglycemic. They can be detected.

Pentamidine can precipitate hypoglycemia, sometimes followed by the onset of diabetes. Its increasingly widespread use in the treatment of intercurrent infections in patients with AIDS requires that considerable caution be exercised.

Management

The drugs can generally be withdrawn and replaced, but behavior modification in a patient with a well-patterned psychiatric disorder is much more difficult.

In diabetics

The use of insulin or sulfonylureas requires knowledge regarding the duration of action of the preparations administered, their potency, and their fate *in vivo*. The hypoglycemias observed in diabetics are a result of one or more of the following causes:

- **Inappropriate prescription**, such as unjustified treatment where diet alone would have been sufficient, or starting the treatment with a loading dose of a potent sulfonylurea that has a long duration of action
- **Renal insufficiency** prolonging the half-life of insulin or sulfonylureas eliminated through the kidney
- **Combination with alcohol** with or without carbohydrate fasting
- **Prescription of a drug potentiating the hypoglycemic effects** of antidiabetic agents. In this connection, it is necessary to consult the current DR (local drug dictionary) for every prescription.

The drugs that have been implicated include principally:

- phenylbutazone and other pyrazolone derivatives
- salicylates (including p-aminosalicylic acid)
- sulfonamides
- coumarin anticoagulants
- beta-blockers
- chloramphenicol
- MAOI
- sympatholytics
  - guanethidine
  - reserpine, clonidine
- miconazole
- clofibrate
- cyclophosphamide
- halofenate
- oxytetracyclines

Certain drug interactions are specific. Tolbutamide metabolic degradation in the liver is diminished by the concomitant administration of **dicoumarol**. Certain antibacterial sulfonamides, sulfamethoxazole and sulfamethoxypyridazine, inhibit the renal excretion of carbutamide and chlorpropamide. Many drugs have a nonspecific competitive interaction for plasma carrier proteins (especially albumin) with sulfonylureas which increase the latter's immediately active free fraction. The risk of an iatrogenic accident increases with the number of drugs coadministered to a patient.

References

Assan R, Girard J, Guillausseau PJ, Lesobre B. Hypoglycémies de l'adulte. In: Tchobroutsky G, Slama G, Assan R, Freychet P, eds. Traité de Diabétologie. Paris: Editions Pradel, 1990: 867–83.

Assan R, Giroud JP, Mathé G, Meyniol G. Insuline et médicaments hypoglycémiants. Pharmacologie Clinique. Bases de la thérapeutique. 2e édition. Paris: Expansion Scientifique Française, 1988: 2288–303.

Bonnefont JP, Specola N, Saudubray JM. Hypoglycémies spontanées de l'enfant. In: Tchobroutsky G, Slama G, Assan R, Freychet P, eds. Traité de Diabétologie. Paris: Editions Pradel, 1990: 884–94.

Chiasson JL, Ekoe JM. Les médicaments modifiant la glycorégulation et les traitements anti-diabétiques. In: Tchobroutsky G, Slama G, Assan R, Freychet P, eds. Traité de Diabétologie. Paris: Editions Pradel, 1990: 741–7.

Seltzer HS. Adverse drug interactions of clinical importance to diabetics. In: Rifkin H, Raskin P, eds. Diabetes Mellitus. Alexandria: American Diabetes Association 1981; 5: 327–34.

Hyperglycemia

With certain substances, the hyperglycemic effect may be part of the desired effects. This is true of glucagon, diazoxide and streptozocin.

Certain other drugs are never used with hyperglycemic intent:

- corticosteroids (administered systemically or topically)
- synthetic estrogens and combinations of estrogens and progestins
- high-dose progestins
- danazol
- L-asparaginase
- diuretics
- beta-agonists
- encainide
- phenytoin
- indomethacin
- azathioprine
- phenothiazines
- pentamidine

Clinically:

- **Beta-agonists** given intravenously to pregnant women can, in a matter of hours, rapidly produce a high level of hyperglycemia together with ketosis, possibly resulting in diabetic coma.
- **Corticosteroids** given systemically are certainly well known as hyperglycemic agents, but it is sometimes overlooked that the administration of topical corticosteroids can be highly diabetogenic, including intra-articular injections of insoluble salts presented as having low diffusion or as nondiffusible. Diabetic decompensation, hyperglycemia and ketosis have been described.

Similarly, long-acting corticosteroids such as sustained-release triamcinolone acetonide can produce bouts of hyperglycemia and ketosis lasting for weeks.

- **Pentamidine**, used increasingly in the treatment of *Pneumocystis carinii* pneumonia, induces hypoglycemia followed by insulin-dependent diabetes.
- **Danazol** can be highly hyperglycemic.

However, any pharmacologic agent deemed necessary must be used, **even** in a diabetic, if there is no alternative.

References

Bouchard P, Sai P, Reach G, et al. Diabetes Mellitus following pentamidine induced hypoglycemia in humans. Diabetes 1982; 31: 405.

Chiasson JL, Ekoe JM. Les médicaments modifiant la glycorégulation et les traitements antidiabétiques. In: Tchobroutsky G, Slama G, Assan R, Freychet P, eds. Traité de Diabétologie. Paris: Editions Pradel, 1990: 741–7.

Tchobroutsky G, Slama G, Chast F. Hyperglycémiants. Pharmacologie Clinique. Bases de la thérapeutique. 2e édition. Paris: Expansion Scientifique Française, 1988: 2305–15.

9 Neurological disorders

Peripheral neuropathy
Pierre Bouche

Definition

Peripheral neuropathy is a general term covering disorders of the principal functions of peripheral nerves, usually related to permanent lesions of the nerve structures or the surrounding interstitial tissue. A contrast exists between primary neurologic causes, most often hereditary, and causes that are secondary to localization of a systemic disease affecting nerves.

Anatomical and clinical forms

According to the site of the predominant elementary lesion, the most frequent forms are axonal neuropathies and demyelinating neuropathies. The differential diagnosis of these two types cannot be effected on the basis of clinical findings; it sometimes requires nerve biopsy, though an electrophysiologic study is generally sufficient.

A pathological process involving the cell body of the peripheral neuron will produce either a motor neuropathy or a sensory neuropathy, also called ganglionopathy.

According to the topography of the clinical manifestations:

- **Polyneuropathy**
  The symptoms are symmetric and predominantly affect the extremities and lower limbs. The polyneuropathy generally begins with sensory disorders consisting of paresthesias, pain or burning sensations, together with motor deficits manifested by stepping gait. Cramps frequently occur. Hypoesthesia in a "stocking" distribution may be accompanied by a loss of position sense. The abolition of tendon reflexes starts with the absence of the Achilles tendon reflexes. The involvement of the upper limbs, predominantly distal, occurs later.

  This is the picture observed most frequently when the cause is toxic or drug-induced. The involvement is generally axonal, with a reduction in the amplitude of sensory and motor evoked potentials. The cerebrospinal fluid is normal.

Adverse Drug Reactions. A Practical Guide to Diagnosis and Management. Edited by C. Bénichou.
©1994 John Wiley & Sons Ltd.

- **Polyradiculoneuritis**
  The lesions are more extensive, affecting the nerve roots, often the entire nerve fiber, and also sometimes the cranial nerves and the nerves supplying the respiratory muscles. Motor disorders are predominant. The acute form of the disease is Guillain–Barré syndrome.

  This category of neuropathy is observed during the course of inflammatory diseases and of immune deficiency disorders. It is a demyelinating neuropathy with slowing of nerve conduction. The cerebrospinal fluid reveals an increase in the protein content without associated pleocytosis.

- **Mononeuropathy multiplex (or mononeuritis)**
  This is characterized by the successive involvement in time and space of several nerve trunks.

Criteria of severity

Immediate

Increasing extension of the paralysis within 2 weeks should raise concern that respiration may become affected, and necessitates intensive monitoring.

Remote

The risk for sequelae is a particular concern when:

- muscular atrophy is severe and widespread
- the distal motor-evoked potentials are reduced in amplitude and profuse fibrillation occurs.

Evidence for a drug-related origin

Drug-induced neuropathy is being identified increasingly. It is sometimes difficult to distinguish it from the complications of the condition being treated (e.g. a paraneoplastic neurological syndrome, diabetic neuropathy). They may be either dose-dependent and appear only after weeks or months, or immunoallergic and appear full-blown within days.

Most drug-induced polyneuropathies are subacute, having an onset of a few weeks or months. Even in these forms, drugs are not the most frequent cause, and one generally begins by ruling out alcohol, diabetes, dysglobulinemia or even a paraneoplastic syndrome before deciding on a drug-related origin. There is no picture that is particularly suggestive of a drug-related etiology.

Time to onset

In the subacute forms, which are the most common, a time frame of a few weeks or a few months is considered to be compatible.

Course

It is considered **suggestive** when the symptoms abate in the months that follow the suspension of the suspect drug, and **compatible** when they do not abate, which generally reflects an extension of the lesions.

Etiologic diagnosis

Possible drug-related causes differ according to the mode of onset and the site of the lesions.

In subacute polyneuropathy (the most common form)

Axonal involvement

A metabolic cause must be considered (diabetes, hypothyroidism, renal insufficiency where the polyneuropathy is usually delayed), association with a nutritional deficiency (vitamins B1, B6, B12, niacin, folates), paraneoplastic syndromes or syndromes secondary to systemic diseases (vasculitis).

Demyelinating forms

These are rarely drug-induced (amiodarone), and must be distinguished from idiopathic inflammatory polyradiculoneuritis or forms secondary to dysglobulinemia or a systemic disease.

Sensory neuropathy may be drug-related (cisplatin, doxorubicin, vitamin B6) and must be distinguished from chronic hereditary forms and subacute paraneoplastic forms.

Acute or chronic polyneuropathy

Acute polyneuropathy, with an onset of less than 4 weeks, or chronic polyneuropathy evolving over several years are not usually associated with drugs.

Drug-related causes

Vinca alkaloids

Vincristine sulfate produces a dose-dependent axonal neuropathy. Vinblastine and vindesine are less toxic.

Cisplatin

The neuropathy is dose-dependent. It affects the spinal ganglion and thus produces an almost pure sensory neuropathy.

Antituberculosis drugs

Isoniazid is the most toxic. The neuropathy is dose-dependent, axonal. Isoniazid interferes with pyridoxine metabolism, which explains the systematic prescription of vitamin B6 when it is used in the treatment of tuberculosis.

Metronidazole

The neuropathy that seems to occur only during prolonged treatment of Crohn's disease is essentially sensory, dose-dependent, axonal.

Disulfiram

This agent, used as an adjunct in alcoholic withdrawal, can induce an axonal, dose-dependent peripheral neuropathy that is difficult to distinguish from alcoholic nutritional neuropathy.

Lithium

The neuropathy appears to develop only with massive doses and reflects acute intoxication. It tends to be a motor neuropathy, similar to Guillain–Barré syndrome, but axonal.

Gold salts

The neuropathy occurs after several months of treatment but has a rapid onset like polyradiculoneuritis, associated with myokimia and mixed axonal-demyelinative lesions. Many authors have concluded that its origin is immunoallergic.

Thalidomide

Thalidomide neuropathy is not uncommon. It is dose-dependent and of the axonal variety.

Amiodarone

The neuropathy generally develops after 1–2 years of treatment at the usual doses. Axonal lesions are frequent, but demyelinative lesions with lysosomal lipid inclusions similar to the ones observed in perhexiline maleate neuropathy have been reported.

Almitrine

The neuropathy occurs after 6 months to a year of treatment, sometimes less. It is dose-dependent and axonal.

Anticoagulants

The neuropathy is generally limited to a single site and is caused by compression from a hematoma in a rigid, unyielding compartment.

Other drugs

Among other reputedly neurotoxic drugs, are nitrofurantoin (only in patients with renal failure), chloroquine (which actually causes neuromyopathy), clioquinol, vidarabine, didanosine, phenytoin, amitriptyline, D-penicillamine, colchicine, dapsone, podophyllin, cimetidine, carbimazole and vitamin B6 (overdose).

Management

A drug-related cause must be considered routinely in any peripheral neuropathy, especially with a subacute form. When the suspicion cannot be dismissed, the treatment must be stopped immediately and clinical and electromyographic surveillance must be instituted, with awareness of the fact that it might take a year for the first signs of recovery to appear. Sometimes, recovery is incomplete and late in occurring. In certain indications, continuation of the treatment is necessary despite the neurologic toxicity.

Certain cases of dose-dependent drug-induced neuropathy can be prevented by adjusting the dosage in patients with renal or hepatic failure.

References

Dicky W, Morrow JI. Drug-induced neurological disorders. Progr Neurobiol 1990; 34: 331–42.

Neau JP, et al. Neuropathies médicamenteuses. Semaine des Hôpitaux de Paris 1987; 63: 3629–35.

Vertigo and associated diseases

Gérard Dordain

Introduction and definitions

The word "vertigo" is often misused by patients and in package inserts to refer, in at least one case out of two, to symptoms that in fact are not related to this disorder of the vestibule of the ear. Vertigo-like symptoms may be due to orthostatic hypotension (often the cause of fainting), cerebellar or proprioceptive disorders, or most frequently to psychological causes such as anxiety attacks with hyperventilation, often referred to as "spasmophilia" or "tetany". Thus, patients should describe exactly what they feel and not only use the word vertigo.

True vertigo is a subjective feeling of mainly rotational movement. A similar sensation is the feeling of displacement especially in connection with movements of the head. Severe rotational vertigo is due to a sudden asymmetrical incongruity between the sensory information reaching the vestibular centers in the brain stem and adjacent structures; the vertigo is thus the result of a sudden unilateral disorder (central or peripheral) of the vestibular nervous system. It is unlikely that a drug would affect only one side of the vestibular system, as systemic drug toxicity cannot be unilateral (unless there is a pre-existent unilateral disorder). Thus, drug-induced vestibular disorders are bilateral and symmetrical and true vertigo, which is caused by a unilateral disorder, cannot be drug-induced.

When an agent that may be potentially harmful to the vestibular system does damage it, the effects are bilateral and simultaneous and there are no localizing signs; this can be seen, for example with too high doses of aminoglycosides. These cases are nearly always irreversible and the clinical picture does not include signs of vestibular laterality: no deviation of the index finger or of the axis of the body or of the gait, and no nystagmus. The patient complains of a very uncomfortable feeling of instability and walks with a drunken gait (apparent on examination). This sensation disappears when still, or when sitting or lying down.

If rotational vertigo is never drug-induced, then the other types of vertigo-like sensations, are more correctly termed feelings of instability, giddiness or dizziness and are almost invariably drug-related. In such cases, it is difficult to locate the origin of these sensations as drugs can affect the vestibular system as well as the cerebellum.

Clinical manifestations

Two rather different situations can arise:

Bilateral vestibular deficit of sudden onset

A bilateral vestibular disorder of sudden or rapid onset (a few hours or days) with neurological deficit that is characterized by nonlateralized static ataxia and drunken gait, both of which will disappear when the patient is sitting or lying down. There is also an absence of signs of vestibular laterality. At most, clinical examination reveals an opsoclonus and, in the severe forms, hypoacusis or bilateral deafness. The clinician may exclude organic disease because of the absence of clinical evidence of vestibular disease but, in fact, the patient's history is the key to the diagnosis, given a previous course of parenteral aminoglycoside administration and confirmation of vestibular damage with total bilateral absence of vestibular reflexes on caloric or rotatory testing. The damage is irreversible, and no treatment is possible except perhaps vestibular re-education which uses nonvestibular pathways with the hope of some compensatory improvement.

Movement-induced dizziness

The second clinical situation is more complicated and concerns the dizziness provoked by head movements, with sometimes postural nystagmus or a slight unsteadiness on standing. The patient may, in addition, present with bilateral tinnitus, and muffled hearing. Clinical examination is unhelpful, and again the history may provide the only clue of the recent (hours or days) introduction of a new drug. Vestibular investigations, when undertaken, show no areflexia in these cases. The clinical course is favorable with a return to normal within a few days of stopping the offending drug.

Signs of severity

Bilateral vestibular areflexia, as revealed by vestibular investigations, is associated with irreversible damage to the sensory vestibular apparatus, more so if there is an additional total bilateral deafness. Renal insufficiency, old age, and the association of several ototoxic drugs increase the risk.

Management

Stopping the offending drug immediately, when possible, is the only way to halt the damage, but even this is often too late with aminoglycosides. If the latter does not apply then recovery will occur within a few days. No drug treatment is available, but re-education of the vestibular system may speed up recovery and avoid stasiphobia.

Mechanism of action

Many drugs can affect the control of balance (vestibular and cerebellar systems), and often may affect hearing. There are no mechanisms or syndromes that are common to these drugs. For example, beta-blockers can induce a bradycardia and reduce the blood flow through a decrease of blood pressure, which is more pronounced when standing. Also, hypoglycemia, toxicity due to alcohol or diphenylhydantoin, or damage of the peripheral apparatus due to high doses of most of the aminoglycosides may be causes. With some drugs, there may be a temporary dysfunction of the cerebellar flocullus shown by nystagmus when the patient is looking deliberately to one side.

DRUGS INDUCING VERTIGO-LIKE SYMPTOMS

Analgesics
dextropropoxyphene*, paracetamol*, pentazocin*

Antibiotics
nalidixic acid*, sulfamethoxazole
aminoglycosides: amikacin, gentamicin, kanamycin, neomycin,
  streptomycin, tobramycin, vancomycin

Antimalarials
chloroquine, quinine

Cardiovascular drugs
beta-blockers*: atenolol, oxprenolol, pindolol, propranolol
vasodilators*: nitrates, nifedipine
antihypertensives*: debrisoquine, methyldopa
digoxin*

Diuretics
ethacrynic acid, clopamide*, cyclopenthiazide*, hydrochlorothiazide

Others: cimetidine*, diazepam, ethinylestradiol*, fenfluramine*,
  indomethacin*, salicylates

*rarely.

Among the aminoglycosides, which are the most toxic, one must separate the different drugs: kanamycin, neomycin and vancomycin, which cause damage to the cochlear apparatus; gentamicin, streptomycin and tobramycin, which affect the vestibular system directly. These antibiotics, when given in overdose, cause irreversible damage to the ciliary cells, otoconial membranes and secretory cells of the inner ear. Toxicity is enhanced by a high peak blood drug level, intravenous injection, renal insufficiency and co-administration of diuretics or antimalarial agents. Dibekacin and ribostamycin appear to be less ototoxic.

The reversible ototoxicity of high-dose salicylate (aspirin) causes bilateral hypoacusis with tinnitus and feelings of drunkenness. Again, a high blood drug level is found but there is no histologic evidence of sensory cell damage, which may explain the reversible nature of the symptoms. Many drugs follow a similar pattern.

Loop diuretics (frusemide and ethacrynic acid) are ototoxic and affect the vascular layer. The lesions are reversible unless aminoglycosides have also been administered.

Alkylating cytotoxic drugs cause irreversible cochlear and vestibular damage.

References

Aumaître O, Vernay D, Courty E, Dordain G. Les médicaments le plus souvent toxiques pour le système nerveux. In: Dehen H, Dordain G, eds. Neuropharmacologie clinique. Paris: Doin, 1989: 536–7.

Brandt Th. Vertigo. Berlin, Heidelberg, New York: Springer Verlag, 1991.

Convulsions

Gérard Dordain

Introduction

Drug-induced convulsions are rare events (0.13% of a cohort of 12,617 patients—Boston Collaborative Drug Surveillance Program 1972); conversely, convulsions following the abrupt withdrawal of a drug are frequent occurrences. In both cases, the drug is only partially responsible for the event, because there are almost always predisposing factors: known epilepsy or an epileptogenic lesion; personal or family history of seizures indicating a low convulsive threshold; interaction with other predisposing drugs or toxic substances (tricyclics, alcohol).

Definition

The convulsions are almost always generalized, of short duration, sometimes repetitive, with a small but real risk of status epilepticus in an at-risk patient such as an alcoholic. When the convulsions are induced by a drug, the interval can be a matter of hours or days, depending on the plasma drug concentration, dosage and method of administration. On the other hand, and more frequently, seizures induced by drug withdrawal occur when the plasma level of the drug is very low. The interval is 24–48 hours for benzodiazepines, the most commonly implicated drug, but may extend to several days, especially when alcohol is withdrawn at the same time.

Features suggestive of a drug-related origin

Two very different situations can be described.

In patients with history of epilepsy

A common cause for the onset of convulsions should be sought: irregular drug administrations (poor compliance is found in around 40% of epileptic patients); alcohol; sleep deprivation or jet lag or similar disturbance in sleeping schedule. In the absence of such causes in a well-controlled patient, any introduction of a new medication must arouse suspicion. The chronology of drug taking should be examined as well as a list of all drugs capable of inducing fits by whatever mechanism (direct toxicity, drug interaction, hypoglycemia, hyperventilation, etc.). See box: *Mechanisms of drug-induced seizures*.

The management of such patients is not clear-cut. It may be useful, first of all, to check the plasma levels of prescribed antiepileptic drugs, knowing that they are less accurate in the case of combination of several drugs. The previous antiepileptic therapy should be reinstated or modified, and clinical outpatient monitoring carried out as a follow-up.

MECHANISMS OF DRUG-INDUCED SEIZURES

Agents that easily cross the blood–brain barrier are those that are most often associated with convulsions, and the risk is even higher with intrathecal administration. Such drugs are, in order of importance, penicillins, insulin and lignocaine.

With semisynthetic penicillins, convulsions are always related to high doses, renal insufficiency or intrathecal administration.

Among phenothiazines, seizures are more often induced by agents with an aliphatic lateral chain (such as chlorpromazine) than by agents with a piperazine chain (such as fluphenazine).

Of the antidepressants, it seems that maprotiline is most risky and should be avoided in epileptic patients. Serotoninergic antidepressants appear to be less epileptogenic than tricyclics.

Mepivacaine and lignocaine cause convulsions when plasma drug levels are excessive, sometimes due to heart failure (by a reduction in the volume of distribution) or to associated hepatic insufficiency.

Slow acetylators are exposed to the risk of convulsions when given isoniazid. Dehydration is a known risk factor with IV contrast medium (metrizamide); risk is increased in patients with intracerebral tumors (gliomas, metastases).

Renal insufficiency also increases the risk of convulsions induced by lithium, nalidixic acid, cimetidine or cephalosporins.

For oxytocin and carbamazepine, convulsions can be explained by prior hyperhydration and/or water intoxication. Chloroquine has a GABA inhibitory action which may explain its capacity to produce convulsions; women appear to be more at risk.

In patients without history of epilepsy

First, the patient history and clinical results should be examined for signs of neurological deficit, leading to confirmatory CT scan. If the clinical examination is negative, a closer investigation into the history might reveal an ill-advised cessation of drug during the hours or days prior to the attack, or other associated risk factors: sleepless nights after running out of benzodiazepine or other medication, alcoholism, which induces seizures on both excessive consumption or withdrawal. When the history has confirmed that the patient has stopped benzodiazepine and alcohol at the same time, which is frequently the case, it would be prudent to request that a CT scan be taken.

BENZODIAZEPINE WITHDRAWAL

> A large-scale epidemiological study concerning the risk factors with benzodiazepine withdrawal (Fialip et al. 1987) has shown that:
>
> Benzodiazepines with short half-lives are not the most frequent cause: all benzodiazepines can cause withdrawal convulsions. Those causing convulsions are simply more widely prescribed.
>
> Neither high doses nor long term treatment increase risk. Seizures have been observed with low doses or short courses of treatment (10 days).
>
> The most important risk factor is the patient himself: known or latent epilepsy, a familial or personal history of epilepsy or childhood convulsions, epileptogenic lesions (trauma sequelae or vascular lesions), concomitant epileptogenic treatment and, most of all, alcoholism.

If the CT scan is negative and drug withdrawal has been established, it is not necessary then to initiate long-term antiepileptic therapy. The benzodiazepine agent can be reinstated and the dose slowly reduced over several weeks, assuming that weaning off the drug is justified.

Signs of severity

In the presence of a severe illness (brain tumor or abscess, septicemia or hemopathy), the onset of seizures after starting a new, essential therapeutic drug can be the cause of many problems, as the new drug may have to be continued despite its known epileptogenic effects or, more often, its interaction with other drugs.

On the other hand, seizures caused by drug withdrawal are more benign, except for the risk of delirium tremens in the alcoholic patient in whom convulsions can also occur.

Table 1 Medications known to cause convulsions

Drugs acting on the CNS
Amphetamines and anorectic agents
Analgesics:
  codeine
  dextropropoxyphene* (overdose)
  pethidine* (mainly in association with phenobarbitone, phenothiazine, tricyclics, MAOIs)
  pentazocine* (overdose)
Anesthetic agents:
  halothane*
  ketamine
  enflurane
  methohexitone (untreated epileptics)
  local anesthetics
Anticholinergic agents:
  orphenadrine
  amantadine*
Anticonvulsants:
  barbiturates (withdrawal)
  phenytoin (overdose)
  carbamazepine (hyperhydration)
Benzodiazepines (withdrawal)
Hypnotic agents:
  methaqualone*
  meprobamate* (withdrawal)
  glutethimide *
Psychotropic agents:
  a) Antidepressants:
      tricyclics and tetracyclics
      MAOIs (in association with tricyclics)
      lithium
  b) Neuroleptics:
      metoclopramide
      phenothiazines (chlorpromazine, prochlorperazine, etc.)
      reserpine and rauwolfia alkaloids
      thioxanthen (chlorproxithen derivatives, flupenthixol)
Others:
  baclofen (withdrawal)
  bemegride
  methylphenidate
  tripelennamine

Antibiotics, antifungal and antiparasitic agents
  amphotericin B
  ampicillin*
  synthetic antimalarials: chloroquine*, pyrimethamine (long-term treatment)
  carbenicillin*
  colistin
  cycloserin*

——————— *continued overleaf*

Table 1   (*continued*)

gentamycin
isoniazid
nalidixic acid* (overdose, renal insufficiency, IV administration)
niridazole
oxacillin
penicillin (renal failure, elderly patients, high doses, IV administration)
polymyxin B
PAS
streptomycin*
sulfonamides
ticarcillin

Chemotherapy agents
actinomycin D*
chlorambucil*
methotrexate
procarbazid
vincristin

Cardiac and respiratory agents
atenolol*
aminophylline
cropropamide and crotethamide*
digitalis derivatives
doxapram*
disopyramide
lignocaine* (IV dose for antiarrythmic properties)
phenylpropanolamine*
podophyllin
propranolol
theophylline (mainly in children)
terbutaline (high doses)

Other drugs
ACTH
aminophenazone (amidopyrine)
bismuth
caffeine
cimetidine* (renal insufficiency)
corticosteroids
desferrioxamine
factor VIII (rapid injection)
folic acid
gallamine
glucagon
gold salts*
indomethacin (in children)
insulin (hypoglycemia)

(*continued*)

Table 1 (*continued*)

levamisole
metrizamide (IV or IT)
naftidrofuryl
phenylbutazone*
probenecid
prostaglandins
vitamin K

*rarely

References

Aumaître O, Vernay D, Courtry E, Dordain G. Les médicaments le plus souvent toxiques pour le système nerveux. In: Dehen H, Dordain G, eds. Neuropharmacologie Clinique. Paris: Doin, 1989; 527–42.

BCDSP (Boston Collaborative Drug Surveillance Program). Drug-induced convulsions, Lancet 1972; ii: 677.

Blain PG, Lane JM. Neurological disorders. In: Davis DM, ed. Textbook of Adverse Drug Reactions. 4th edition. Oxford: Oxford University Press, 1991; 524–66.

Fialip J, Aumaître O, Eschalier A, Maradeix B, Dordain G, Lavarenne J. Benzodiazepine withdrawal seizures: analysis of 48 case reports. Clinical Neuropharmacology 1987; 10, 6: 538–544.

Muscular disorders

Didier Vernay

Introduction

Drug-induced myopathies are relatively common. However, the existence of drug-induced muscle weakness, myalgia or cramps is not well known and therefore the relationship is only rarely recognized. Severe reactions such as rhabdomyolysis with acute renal failure have been described, but the clinical features are generally moderate and the symptoms begin to subside as soon as the drug is stopped.

Muscle disorders can be caused by a number of different mechanisms, genetic (myopathies), toxic, metabolic and inflammatory (polymyositis), but the clinical presentations are often similar: symmetrical and often proximal distribution of the motor deficit with an acute or progressive onset and the presence or absence of pain.

The exact mechanism of drug-induced muscle disorders is unknown in most cases. In some cases a metabolic factor may appear to be an important factor; in other cases, an immune mechanism appears to be more likely.

In cases of toxic myopathies there are in addition to the clinical presentation raised levels of muscle cell enzymes (CPK), **electromyographic (EMG) changes**, i.e. "myogenic" signs (small, short-lived, polyphasic potentials of low amplitude), and a **histological** picture of necrotic areas and sometimes vacuoles.

Drug-induced myopathies may be classified as those **with** and those **without pain,** and further subdivided according to the presence or absence of neurological signs or symptoms. In addition, **disorders of neuromuscular transmission** (myasthenic syndromes), **malignant hyperthermia, myotonic reactions** and **focal muscle disorders** will be described.

At the end of this section, Table 2 summarizes the **various drugs associated with these different myopathies.**

Clinical classification

Painless myopathies

Myopathies without neuropathy

Chronic **corticosteroid** therapy is most often the cause of this group of myopathies. There are many subclinical forms, as well as those associated with the disease for which the drugs were prescribed, for example a polymyositis or a systemic autoimmune disease (rheumatoid arthritis, systemic lupus erythematosus). All corticosteroids can induce these disorders, but especially the fluorinated compounds (triamcinolone, betamethasone, dexamethasone).

The onset is usually progressive and affects axial and proximal muscles. Neck flexor muscles tend not to be affected by corticosteroid-induced myopathies, which might help the differential diagnosis with a polymyositis. Levels of CPK are not raised, but urinary creatinine is raised, in proportion to the severity of the muscle deficit. The deficit occurs from 4 to 32 weeks after starting therapy and is not clearly dose-dependent; however, the deficit usually diminishes on a significant reduction in dosage, or on stopping the drug.

Beta-blockers such as sotalol and propranolol can also induce this type of myopathy.

Myopathies with neuropathy

Colchicine can produce a neurological and muscle disorder with proximal muscle weakness, distal areflexia and a mild distal sensory deficit. Muscle cell enzyme levels are invariably raised. The main risk factor in such cases is chronic renal failure.

Chloroquine and **hydroxychloroquine** have also been implicated, presenting with a relatively specific weakness of the scapular muscles. Associated diseases include heart failure and degenerative retinal lesions.

Painful myopathies

Painful polymyositis-type myopathies

D-penicillamine can induce this type of myopathy. A dermatopolymyositis-like rash and dysphagia are common presentations. Cardiac involvement is rare but may require instituting steroid therapy. Other drugs include thiol compounds (tiopronine, pirithioxine).

Zidovudine (AZT) can pose an additional problem in the differential diagnosis of an HIV-induced myopathy. However, the drug-induced myopathy is usually subacute, with an insidious onset. The lower limbs are preferentially affected, and are painful on palpation. The differentiating feature is that HIV-induced myopathy is usually painless. Levels of CPK are raised in AZT myopathies but normal in those caused by HIV.

Painful nonpolymyositis-type myopathies

Many drugs are associated with this group of muscle disorders, in particular the **lipid-lowering drugs** (fibrate, lovastatin, simvastatin, gemfibrozil) due to their rapidly increasing sales. Fibrate-induced myopathies can develop within 2 days to 2 years of treatment, particularly in the presence of renal failure and hypothyroidism. The accumulated effects of the various lipid-lowering drugs, particularly as a result of overlapping in drug therapies, can lead to drug-induced problems. Monitoring of creatine kinase levels appears to be insufficient to avoid the occurrence of these complications.

Cyclosporin has induced generalized muscle pain and cramps associated with asthenia in some patients. Creatine kinase levels were raised whilst the drug concentrations remained within the therapeutic range. Most cases were associated with renal insufficiency with cyclosporin being administered concomitantly with other myotoxic drugs. Numerous case reports suggest a cumulative toxicity in such cases.

Painful myopathies with neuropathy

Vincristine is a well-known cause of cumulative toxicity and can induce painful proximal muscle weakness with amyotrophy.

Amiodarone can also produce a predominant neuropathy. **Hypokalemic agents** (diuretics, laxatives, liquorice) can lead to proximal muscle deficits with pain and areflexia. Laboratory tests often reveal hypochloremic alkalosis with hypokalemia (<2 mmol/L). Symptoms such as dysphoria and hallucinations may occur.
Hypophosphatemic agents (long-term antacid therapy, prolonged 5% dextrose infusions) cause similar clinical syndromes.

Rhabdomyolysis

Some of the drugs that can induce painful myopathies and/or some toxic agents can also cause necrotizing myopathies with associated myoglobinuria and renal failure. Drug abuse with opioids, amphetamines or alcohol is often responsible, with a background of generalized weakness. The onset is acute, with intensely painful muscles. Areflexia may occur, as well as acute renal failure due to tubular necrosis. Central neurological signs can aggravate the clinical picture with confusion, convulsions and even coma. Admission to an intensive care unit is essential in cases of acute renal failure.

A syndrome associating **myalgia** and **hypereosinophilia** has been reported with the use of **tryptophan**. This aminoacid has been prescribed in the treatment of insomnia, depression and premenstrual syndrome. The onset of the syndrome is abrupt with malaise, myalgia and a muscle weakness associated with a sensation of induration or contracture of the fascia. Associated cutaneous reactions have been reported that resemble scleroderma or an urticarial rash. ESR and blood creatinine levels are normal, but serum aldolase levels are raised. Other systemic disorders, including pulmonary or pleural, cardiac, rheumatological, digestive or oral, may be seen. The Center for Disease Control in the USA has described the following diagnostic criteria: eosinophilia of $>10^9$ cells/L, crippling myalgia and diagnostic exclusion of infection or malignant disease as a cause.

Despite stopping the drug, symptoms may persist or even worsen in some cases. Corticosteroid therapy at 30–60 mg/day is necessary in the majority of these patients. An excipient or cofactors (bacitracin-like peptides) could be involved as the etiological agents of these disorders.

Other iatrogenic disorders affecting muscle function

Myasthenic syndromes (anomalies of neuromuscular transmission)

Many drugs can cause a myasthenic syndrome, or aggravate or reveal a pre-existing syndrome. **Penicillamine** is the most frequent inducer of the myasthenic syndrome. The clinical picture is that of myasthenia gravis with oculomotor symptoms, and bulbar or limb palsies that are aggravated by effort and improved by rest. Postoperative apnea may also occur. Serum levels of muscular enzymes remain normal, and EMG reveals a progressive reduction in action potentials on repetitive stimulation. Antiacetylcholine receptor antibodies may be found. Anticholinesterase therapy may be effective.

Myotonic reactions

Myotonia is defined by a delayed relaxation of the muscles after contraction. This is characteristic of some congenital syndromes (Steinert's and Thomsen's diseases). The drugs that may produce such clinical and electromyographic consequences include suxamethonium, propranolol, 20-25 diazacholesterol, clofibrate and nifedipine.

Malignant hyperthermia

Malignant hyperthermia is a severe, sometimes fatal complication of the use of anesthetic agents. There is a genetic predisposition in certain patients who have raised CPK levels, but this is a poor predictor. Some patients who develop this disorder may have previous and uneventful exposure to anesthetic agents.

The drugs most frequently implicated include **halothane** and **suxamethonium**. The hyperthermia may occur during the administration of anesthesia or shortly after. The hyperthermia is severe, with metabolic acidosis, diffuse muscular rigidity and myoglobinuria. The specific treatment consists of an immediate intravenous infusion of dantrolene. Malignant hyperthermia can also be induced by tricyclic antidepressants and MAOIs.

Suxamethonium-induced postoperative myalgias are common occurrences and can be prevented by preoperative administration of 600 mg of aspirin.

Focal myopathies

These are rare occurrences, but repeated IM injections can in themselves induce rises in CPK levels, and may include induration and muscle contractures. The most likely causative drugs are pentazocine, meperidine, chloroquine, opioids, chlorpromazine and phenytoin. Antibiotics have also been implicated, in children in particular, in whom extensive fibrosis may occur after long-term treatment.

Conclusion

When presented with a clinical picture including proximal muscle weakness, with or without myalgia, a drug-related etiology should be considered. In the vast majority of cases, stopping the drug treatment results in rapid resolution of the signs and symptoms. It is important to bear in mind, when prescribing further treatments, that the presence of renal or hepatic insufficiency or concomitant cyclosporin therapy may increase the risk of drug-induced myopathy.

References

Aumaître O, Vernay D, Courtry E, Dordain G. Les médicaments le plus souvent toxiques pour le système nerveux. In: Dehen H, Dordain G, eds. Neuropharmacologie Clinique. Paris: Doin, 1989: 527–42.

Blain PG, Lane JM. Neurological disorders. In: Davis DM, ed. Textbook of Adverse Drug Reactions. 4th edition. Oxford: Oxford University Press, 1991: 524–66.

Le Quintrec JS, Le Quintrec JL. Drug-induced myopathies. Baillière's Clinical Rheumatology. 1991; 1, 5: 21–38.

Table 2 Principal drugs causing muscular disorders

Painless myopathies
Painless myopathies without neuropathy
- corticosteroids
- beta-blockers

Painless myopathies without neuropathy
- colchicine
- chloroquine, hydroxychloroquine
- perhexiline maleate

Painful myopathies
Painful polymyositis (polymyositis type)
- D-penicillamine and thiol derivatives
- zidovudine
- cimetidine
- penicillin, sulfonamide
- phenylbutazone, niflumic acid
- propylthiouracil
- hydralazine, procainamide
- cocaine

Painful myopathies (nonpolymyositis type)
- hypolipemic agents: fibrates, statins
- cyclosporin
- quinolones, nalidixic acid
- enalapril
- emetine, carbimazole
- etretinate
- sodium cromoglycate
- minoxidil
- aminocaproic acid
- metoprolol
- suxamethonium

Painful myopathies with neuropathy
- vincristine
- amiodarone
- hypokalamic agents
- hypophosphatemic agents

Rhabdomyolysis
- alcohol, heroin, amphetamines, caffeine
- phencyclidine
- aspirin

Hypereosinophilic myalgic syndrome
- L-tryptophan

Iagtrogenic disorders affecting muscular function
Myasthenic syndrome
- D-penicillamine and thiol derivatives

continued overleaf

Table 2   (*continued*)

- chloroquine
- antibiotics (aminoglycosides + +)
- beta-blockers

Myotonic reaction
- suxamethonium
- propranolol
- 20-25 diazacholesterol

Malignant hyperthermia
- anesthetics (halothane, suxamethonium)
- tricyclic antidepressants, MAOIs

Focal myopathy
- pentazocine
- meperidine
- chloroquine
- opioids
- chlorpromazine
- phenytoin
- antibiotics

Source: after Le Quintrec and Le Quintrec 1991.

Extrapyramidal disorders

Didier Deffond

Parkinsonian syndromes

Definition and etiology

A parkinsonian syndrome involves (with some variations) plastic rigidity, delay in initiating movements (akinesia), a slowing down of voluntary activity with possible loss of some automatic movements (bradykinesia) and, finally, a resting and/or postural tremor.

Etiology

This triple combination defines Parkinson's disease, but it will be seen in other degenerative diseases of the basal ganglia (these are currently amalgamated under the heading of "multisystem atrophy" or "MSA"). A common feature of these disorders involves a lesion of the nigrostriatal dopaminergic pathway. A number of drugs are also capable of provoking a parkinsonian syndrome.

Drugs involved

The neuroleptics, because of their mechanism of action, which blocks the dopaminergic receptors, are the drugs most commonly responsible. The incidence of the parkinsonian syndrome after prolonged treatment with a neuroleptic drug is 20%. Reserpine and tetrabenazine, which deplete the presynaptic dopamine synapses, are rarely used now but induce a parkinsonian syndrome very frequently.

The risk is increased with a higher dose, increasing age, and in female subjects.

All the neuroleptic drugs are involved regardless of their chemical class. Amoxapine, a neuroleptic derivative with antidepressant action, is also frequently involved. Parkinsonian syndromes have also been described after prolonged calcium inhibitor therapy, such as flunarizine and cinnarizine. The regression of the symptoms is as slow as with the neuroleptics. A worsening of the extrapyramidal symptoms has been described in a few cases with tricyclic antidepressants and fluoxetine (nontricyclic antidepressant). An akinetic rigid syndrome can also be induced by the antihypertensive drug alpha-methyldopa, most likely due to its competition with dopamine.

Children can also develop, exceptionally, a parkinsonian syndrome induced by chloroquine and amodiaquine.

Evidence implicating a drug

Chronology

A neuroleptic-induced parkinsonian syndrome appears shortly after the beginning of the treatment, from a few days to a few weeks, rarely after three months.

Clinical features

There are three main characteristics of a drug-induced syndrome:

- a symmetrical distribution; idiopathic Parkinson's disease starts and predominates in most cases in one half of the body;
- a tremor, if present, is more likely to be postural in type (essential tremor) than resting tremor;
- the existence of a buccofacial dyskinesia which is never seen in untreated parkinsonian disease. This is the only absolute criteria, because a postneuroleptic-induced syndrome may, except for this sign, be indistinguishable from an idiopathic disease.

Management

A variety of drugs has been prescribed to correct neuroleptic-induced extrapyramidal syndrome, such as anticholinergics and amantadine. Their beneficial effects are weak and they have significant side-effects of their own. High dosages of levodopa may be useful, but increase the risk of buccofacial dyskinesia and of reactivation of delusions in psychosis.

The only effective measure is to reduce the dose of the drug to an absolute minimum, or stop the drug if at all possible. The parkinsonian syndrome will disappear slowly, completely after several months. If the syndrome persists after a year, it may just have been idiopathic Parkinson's disease unmasked by the neuroleptics.

References

Bouchard RH, Pourcher E, Vincent P. Fluoxetine and extrapyramidal side effects. Am J Psychiatry 1989; 146: 1352–3.

Micheli F, Pardal MF, Gatto M, Torres M, Paradiso G, Parera IC, Giannalva R. Flunarizine- and cinnarizine-induced extrapyramidal reactions. Neurology 1987; 37: 881–4.

Tarsy C. Neuroleptics-induced extrapyramidal reactions: classification, description and diagnosis. Clinical Neuropharmacology 1987; 6: 527–34.

Abnormal movements

Didier Deffond

Definitions

Tremor

A tremor is defined as a rhythmic oscillation of all or part of the body around its position of equilibrium. The movement is produced by an alternating contraction of agonist and antagonist muscles.

Clinically, three types of tremor are described, depending on the circumstance of their occurrence: at rest, postural and intentional (induced during a voluntary movement).

Chorea

This is involuntary, irregular, rapid, asymmetric, unpredictable, nonstereotyped movement, involving any part of the body, but mostly the extremities or the face. It occurs at rest but can also disturb voluntary movement.

Ballismus is a clinical variation of chorea that affects the proximal muscles of the limbs resulting in violent, flinging movements.

Dystonia

Dystonic movement is due to involuntary, prolonged muscular contractions of individual muscles or muscle groups, leading to an abnormal posture of a limb, a part of a limb or axis of the body. The distribution is more often proximal and axial. Dystonia of the extremities is sometimes called athetosis.

Dystonic movements are stereotyped for an individual patient, triggered and/or aggravated by voluntary movement.

Akathisia

A voluntary movement induced by a compulsive need for the patient to move. The movements are often stereotyped, marching on the spot or constant crossing and uncrossing of the legs in the sitting position. The mood is almost always elated.

Dyskinesia

Dyskinesia is a synonym for abnormal movement, so that all the movements described above are dyskinetic. This word is often used for drug-induced reactions, which reflect the heterogeneity of the signs involved.

Tremor

This is generally considered as an exaggeration of the physiological tremor. The frequency is therefore high (8–12 Hz), and the tremor is postural. Its amplitude can be as high as several centimeters, creating severe impairment of function. The principal drugs involved are sodium valproate, lithium, tricyclic antidepressants, sympathomimetics and theophylline. When the tremor due to these drugs is disabling, it is usually possible to change the drug for another one of similar efficacy, e.g. another antiepileptic instead of sodium valproate, carbamazepine for lithium, etc.

Acute neuroleptic dyskinesia

The abnormal movements appear within 4 days of starting a neuroleptic treatment or when increasing the dose in cases of a long-term treatment. Clinically they include mainly dystonic reactions involving neck and face. Younger patients are more at risk, and the younger the patient is the more likely is the dystonia to be generalized. In children, a pseudotetanic picture with trismus and opisthotonos can occur.

These acute dystonias disappear in a few hours or days after stopping the drug, or sometimes even if the treatment is continued (tolerance phenomena). IV anticholinergic agents have a dramatic curative effect in a few minutes. Anticholinergics can be used prophylactically in patients at risk (younger than 40), but the duration of the latter treatment should be no more than 2 weeks, because of the increased risk of tardive dyskinesia.

Tardive dyskinesia

A variety of abnormal movements are also seen in tardive dyskinesia but almost always comprise "choreodystonic" movements involving the face and mouth, as well as pure limb or axial dystonia (sometimes mimicking spasmodic torticollis).

Tardive akathisia is often also a feature. Severe buccofacial dyskinesia can cause dyspnea and lethal aspiration pneumonia. Tardive dyskinesia appears after at least 3 months of treatment by neuroleptic drugs. After 5 years, 30% of patients are affected to a greater or lesser extent. These abnormal movements can occur spontaneously in some schizophrenic patients, especially those said to be "deficient."

After stopping the drug, the symptoms tend to worsen and then slowly improve in a matter of months or even years, in 70% of cases. In 30% of cases, the dyskinesia becomes permanent.

Elderly and female patients are more at risk, and are also less likely to improve after stopping the drug. Caution should be exercised when prescribing neuroleptics in this group of patients, particularly those with a non psychiatric indication, such as metoclopramide in gastroenterology or neuroleptic drugs marketed as "hypnotics."

Diltiazem and buspirone have been used as curative treatments with partial and variable results. Reserpine or tetrabenazine can be used successfully but may induce a parkinsonian syndrome or depression. The anticholinergic drugs are contraindicated as they can aggravate the symptoms.

Dopaminergic-induced dyskinesia

In patients treated for idiopathic Parkinson's disease, and only in those patients, levodopa induces, almost constantly, "choreodystonic" movements after some months or years of treatment. After 5 years' treatment with L-dopa, 90% of patients will suffer from more or less severe dyskinesias. In monotherapy, the direct dopamine agonists (bromocriptine, lisuride, pergolide, piribedil), seem less frequently involved. The dyskinesias appearing (the so-called "peak dose" dyskinesias) are usually only slightly disabling even if they sometimes look spectacular. These have to be distinguished from those occurring at the beginning and end of the dose interval (the so-called "beginning and end of dose" or "biphasic" dyskinesias). Their dystonic nature often makes them painful, this and their throwing-type movements producing a severe functional impairment.

Other drug-induced dyskinesias

Choreiform syndromes often affecting only half of the body have been occasionally described in young women on oral contraceptives after a few months of treatment. Most patients had a previous history of Sydenham's chorea or rheumatic fever. Rapid and complete resolution of the symptoms occurs after stopping the drug.

Phenytoin can on rare occasions induce a diffuse reversible "choreodystonic" syndrome, especially in patients with intracerebral lesions. Isolated cases of dyskinesias due to other anticonvulsants have been reported, but only due to overdosage. Anecdotal reports of choreiform syndromes induced by amphetamines, pemoline, cimetidine and tricyclics (after neuroleptic pretreatment) have been published.

References

Harrison MB, Lyons GR, Landow ER. Phenytoin and dyskinesias: a report of two cases and review of the literature. Movement Disorders 1993; 8: 19–27.

Jenner P, Marsden CD. Neuroleptics and tardive dyskinesia. In: Coyle JY, Enna SJ, eds. Neuroleptics: Neurochemical Behavioral and Clinical Perspectives. New York: Raven Press, 1983: 223–253.

Leys D, Destee A, Petit H, Warot P. Chorea associated with oral contraception. J Neurol 1987; 235: 46–8.

10 Abnormal blood pressure

Hypotension
Catherine Chapelon

Drug-induced hypotension may be persistent or postural, as in the case of orthostatic hypotension. (*Acute hypotension associated with anaphylactic reactions is discussed elsewhere.*)

It is difficult to set a lower limit for the systolic blood pressure (BP) level defining hypotension. The diagnosis should be based on a change from the previous BP measurement, especially if it is accompanied by a sense of malaise, dizziness or, of course, loss of consciousness.

Elderly patients should be screened regularly for a marked drop in BP which may be poorly tolerated and can be responsible for serious complications such as coronary insufficiency, cerebrovascular accident or faintness that may bring on a fall and a consequent fracture.

Causative drugs

Any antihypertensive drug may be involved; the problem is more one of adjustment to dosage rather than an adverse reaction.

With some medications, and particularly certain vasodilators, hypotension is most likely to occur at the beginning of administration. In the case of long-standing treatment, look for a contributory factor, in particular sodium depletion (dietary restriction, diarrhea, etc.).

Drugs belonging to other therapeutic classes can produce a drop in blood pressure that may or may not be accompanied by clinical symptoms.

They include antipsychotic drugs (phenothiazine derivatives or others), tricyclic antidepressants (e.g. imipramine), MAOIs, quinidine antiarrhythmic agents and nitrates.

Adverse Drug Reactions. A Practical Guide to Diagnosis and Management. Edited by C. Bénichou.
©1994 John Wiley & Sons Ltd.

Management

In elderly patients, hypotension accompanied by a feeling of malaise or dizziness calls for discontinuation of the treatment because of the risk of complications. In the absence of severe symptoms, a decrease in dosage may be sufficient. In all cases, should hypovolemia occur, it must be corrected.

Orthostatic hypotension

Catherine Chapelon

Definition

This is a fall in systolic BP of more than 20 mmHg on rising from a recumbent position.

Orthostatic hypotension stimulates the aortic and carotid baroreceptors, which in turn activate the vasomotor and cardioaccelerating centers, producing reflex vasoconstriction and accelerating the heart rate.

The clinical signs are the same as in chronic hypotension but they occur only when the upright position is assumed. The cardiovascular consequences are comparable.

Etiology

Drugs occupy an important place in the etiology of orthostatic hypotension, which is then accompanied almost invariably by tachycardia, except when caused by agents that produce bradycardia.

The other principal causes include brain tumors and degenerative central nervous system diseases. A dysfunction of the reflex arc of baroreceptors can be observed in certain carotid sinus lesions (atheroma, cervical radiotherapy), trauma to the spine, degenerative myelopathies or demyelinating diseases of the spinal cord and nerves, extensive sympathectomy, porphyria and amyloidosis.

The causative drugs are:

- all antihypertensive drugs
- agents that act on the baroreceptor reflex arc: tranquillizers, sedatives or hypnotics, antidepressants.

Management

In symptomatic elderly patients, the treatment must be stopped in a more or less gradual way, depending on each medication. In some cases, hospitalization may be necessary. If orthostatic hypotension is discovered by chance, the dosage should be reduced and, if necessary, this should be accompanied by simple measures (gradual rising from the supine position, elastic supportive hose around the calves) to permit continuation of the treatment.

Hypertension

Eugène Rothschild

Definition

Arterial hypertension is defined as BP more than 160/90 mmHg in adults of 18 years or older.

Drug-induced hypertension

Drug-induced hypertension is a result of the pharmacologic mode of action of the causative agents. Their site of action on the BP-regulating mechanisms (sodium balance, vascular tone, central nervous system) varies with the individual drug. Even though this type of reaction is predictable, hypertension does not occur in all patients who are treated.

Hypertension may also be a symptom of drug-induced nephropathy that requires a different approach.

- **The incidence of drug-induced hypertension varies greatly with the causative agent.** For example:
  - With cyclosporin, the frequency of induced hypertension is as high as 60% or even 95% in some series of organ transplantation.
  - Recombinant erythropoietin produces hypertension in an average of 30% of patients on dialysis.
  - Oral contraceptives (but not transdermal estrogens) regularly produce a moderate increase in BP, though hypertension occurs in less than 5% of the women treated.

*In treated hypertensive patients, **certain drug interactions** can reduce the effectiveness of the antihypertensive treatment. For example:*

- ***NSAIDs** can antagonize a number of antihypertensive agents (diuretics, beta-blockers, converting enzyme inhibitors), but do not do so consistently.*
- ***Alpha-sympatholytics**, like tricyclic antidepressants and phenothiazines, can inhibit drugs that have a central antihypertensive action.*
- ***Sympathomimetics** may **acutely aggravate** hypertension in patients treated with beta-blocking agents or centrally acting antihypertensives.*

— With phenylpropanolamine, such cases are rare, at least at the usual doses, in normotensive individuals.

- *Pharmacokinetic interactions* may reduce the bioavailability of certain antihypertensives (for example, enzyme inducers and beta-blockers that undergo extensive hepatic first-pass metabolism).

- The factors accounting for individual susceptibility to the hypertensive effect of certain drugs are often poorly understood. However, some **contributing factors** have been identified:

  — an *excessive dose*: sympathomimetics (nasal decongestants, appetite suppressants, etc.), cyclosporin, glycyrrhizic acid, (derivatives of licorice);

  — a *drug interaction*: certain interactions can potentiate the effect of pressor substances; for example, BP elevations (sometimes considerable) can be induced by the simultaneous administration of phenylpropanolamine and NSAIDs or MAOIs.

  Certain agents that have no hypertensive effect by themselves may induce hypertension when combined with other drugs, such as MAOIs and antihistamines, oxytocics and ergot alkaloids.

  — *diet* can be a factor. A sodium-rich diet promotes hypertension induced by mineralocorticoids (but not by glucocorticoids) and facilitates the inhibitory effect of NSAIDs on antihypertensive action.

  Foods rich in tyrosine can precipitate hypertensive crises in patients treated with MAOIs.

  — *underlying conditions*: in patients with chronic renal failure, hypertension is induced more easily by certain agents (e.g. glucocorticoids, recombinant erythropoietin, cyclosporin).

  In pheochromocytoma, dopamine antagonists (sulpiride, metoclopramide) may precipitate bouts of hypertension.

Diagnosis

The diagnostic problem arises in various settings

The **onset of hypertension** in a previously normotensive patient must systematically trigger inquiry into drug use, to identify a drug liable to produce a pressor effect.

A complete etiologic investigation must be conducted, bearing in mind that a cause (sometimes rectifiable) is found in only about 5% of the hypertensive patients.

A **hypertensive patient whose BP is no longer controlled** by the treatment must also be questioned systematically about the drugs he or she is taking, including agents that might interact with antihypertensives.

Watch out for the following:

- *an overlooked cause of secondary hypertension such as renal artery stenosis*
- *poor antihypertensive treatment compliance*
- *improper use of antihypertensive drugs: for example, clonidine administered intravenously or in combination with a beta-blocking agent may aggravate hypertension; a hypertensive bout may occur following abrupt discontinuation (sometimes unintentional) of certain centrally acting antihypertensives or the prescription of beta-blockers to patients with pheochromocytoma.*

When a drug, **the possible hypertensive effect of which is known, is prescribed,** good medical practice calls for routine monitoring of BP.

In all cases, be aware that:

- *Spontaneous variability is one of the characteristics of BP.*
- *Exercise, pain, emotion, stress, etc., will elevate BP; bouts of hypertension can be observed in association with a cerebrovascular accident, acute pulmonary edema, but also with epistaxis, simple headache, etc.*

Diagnostic criteria

There is no criterion for the drug-induced origin of hypertension

- There is no symptomatologic (clinical) criterion: there is a vast range of possible manifestations, from a moderate BP elevation to causing an immediate large rise which is dangerous (grade III or IV fundus) or complicated (cerebrovascular accident, acute pulmonary edema).
- There is no temporal criterion: the timing of the onset and of abatement on stopping treatment is variable from one class of drugs to the next (from an immediate effect to a period of several months); however, for a given agent, the time-lag to onset and to resolution is of the same extent.

Diagnostic considerations
The diagnosis of drug-induced hypertension is based on:

- *a return to the previous BP levels when the drug is withdrawn (but that does not constitute unfailing evidence, given the variability of BP)*
- *the characteristics of the pharmacologic agent and, in particular:*
  - *prevalence of hypertension in treated patients*
  - *known plausible physiopathologic mechanisms*
  - *presence of validated contributing circumstances, if any*
  - *lack of plausible alternative explanations.*

Management

It depends on the following:

- expected therapeutic benefits of the implicated drug
- scheduled duration of the treatment
- degree of blood pressure elevation induced.

The simplest course is to withdraw the suspect drug and monitor the BP.

Emergency hospitalization may be necessary if the patient is in immediate danger as a result of the acute hypertension or, to an even greater extent, there is serious organ damage.

However, continuation of the treatment may be justified when:

- hypertension remains moderate and the causative treatment is prescribed for a short period of time;

- there is a compelling need for the drug implicated (for example, erythropoietin, cyclosporin) and the hypertension is amenable to simple therapeutic measures (reduction in dosage of the involved drug, salt-free diet, effective change in antihypertensive treatment).

References

Grünfeld JP, Bellet M. À propos des hypertensions artérielles induites par les médicaments. Nephrologie 1982; 3: 167–70.

Lai KN, Richards AM, Nicholls MG. Drug-induced hypertension. Adverse Drug React Toxicol Rev 1991; 10: 31–46.

11 Cardiac disorders

Arrhythmia in an antiarrhythmic drug-treated patient

Jacques Caron

Certain drugs may be responsible for proarrhythmic (arrhythmogenic) effects that can have dramatic consequences. This type of adverse reaction is particularly confusing and paradoxical with antiarrhythmic drugs that sometimes produce just the opposite of the desired result. This problem of proarrhythmic effects will be discussed here only as it relates to antiarrhythmic drugs, though it should be noted that other drugs may also cause this adverse reaction, notably certain cardiotonics or psychotropic agents.

Definition

In a patient treated with an antiarrhythmic drug, a proarrhythmic effect must be considered in the presence of:

- aggravation of a pre-existing arrhythmia
- occurrence of a new rhythm disorder.

It is difficult to estimate the incidence of proarrhythmic effects of antiarrhythmic drugs. Above all, it varies greatly according to the agents involved, the clinical conditions and the criteria that are used to judge proarrhythmic drug effects.

An average incidence of about 11% has been described and is often cited. The difficulty in interpreting figures given in the literature should be emphasized.

Mechanisms

These are not completely clear. Besides the mechanisms involving enhanced automaticity (whose exact significance remains to be precisely clarified), two

A conduction disorder may worsen or may create (de novo) reentry, which is known to play an important part in producing ventricular arrhythmia

Adverse Drug Reactions. A Practical Guide to Diagnosis and Management. Edited by C. Bénichou.
©1994 John Wiley & Sons Ltd.

mechanisms have been clearly identified as potentially responsible for initiating arrhythmia:

- Aggravation or onset of a conduction disorder

(especially at the chronic stage of myocardial infarction).

- Triggering of afterdepolarizations at the cellular level, which itself can produce trigger activity.

Early afterdepolarizations (occurring prior to the end of cell depolarization) could be the cause of torsade de pointes.

Arrhythmias suggesting a proarrhythmic drug effect

Supraventricular proarrhythmic effects

- Acceleration of the ventricular rate, enhanced ventricular response to atrial flutter or to atrial tachycardia (AT)

This adverse reaction may be linked to:

- *sufficient slowing of the atrial rate in a patient with arrhythmia to permit the atrioventricular node to recover from its refractory period and thus increase the ventricular rate. As an example, an AT with a rate of 250 beats/min transmitted to the ventricles during a 2:1 block of AV conduction (ventricular rate of 125/min) may be slowed to 200 beats/min by an antiarrhythmic treatment and will then be transmitted to the ventricles at a rate of 1:1 with a ventricular rate of 200 beats/min.*
- *The anticholinergic effect of certain antiarrhythmic agents (disopyramide) that can facilitate atrioventricular conduction.*

- Enhanced ventricular response to atrial fibrillation complicating a Wolf–Parkinson–White syndrome (accessory pathway bypassing the atrioventricular node)

This proarrhythmic effect is produced by digitalis glycosides (or certain calcium antagonists) which shorten the accessory pathway's refractory period and slow conduction in the atrioventricular node, allowing a massive passage of impulses through the accessory pathway and exposing the patient to the risk of an extremely rapid tachyarrhythmia.

- Aggravation of junctional tachycardia which, in its most severe form, consists of incessant junctional tachycardia.

This is an uncommon event, related in particular to the use of class I antiarrhythmic agents, especially the most potent ones (class Ic).

Ventricular proarrhythmic effects

- Aggravation of a pre-existing arrhythmia:
- by increasing the number of premature beats
- by increasing the number of premature beats occurring in runs
- by worsening a nonsustained (< 30 seconds) or sustained (> 30 seconds) ventricular tachycardia.

An increase in the number of ventricular premature beats or runs of extrasystoles poses two problems that are difficult to interpret:

- *the spontaneous variability of an arrhythmia may actually "mimic" a proarrhythmic effect*
- *the spontaneous course of an underlying cardiopathy may itself aggravate an arrhythmia.*

It has also been established that the milder the initial (pretreatment) arrhythmia (quantitatively speaking), the more severe the aggravation must be before it can be classified as a proarrhythmic drug effect.

- Onset of a new ventricular arrhythmia:
- sustained ventricular tachycardia (or ventricular fibrillation)

A definite diagnosis of proarrhythmic effect is contingent upon the onset, shortly after institution of the treatment or a dosage increment, of an incessant ventricular tachycardia that is refractory to programmed ventricular stimulation or cardioversion or is immediately relapsing and ceases only on discontinuation of the drug.

In other cases, a body of evidence may be used to link the arrhythmia to a proarrhythmic effect (see later).

- Torsades de pointes episodes are usually drug-induced.

Antiarrhythmic agents play a large part in the etiology of torsades de pointes:

- *class I (especially Ia) antiarrhythmic agents*
- *sotalol*
- *amiodarone*
- *bepridil.*

Evidence for a proarrhythmic drug effect at the ventricular level

Aggravation of a pre-existing arrhythmia

The only strong evidence is a return of the arrhythmia to its initial level without any change being made other than to withdraw the suspect drug.

One should take into account not only the elimination time of the drug but also that of its active metabolites.

In the aggravation of a severe arrhythmia (ventricular tachycardia), this evidence is usually unavailable because of the necessity to manage the proarrhythmic effect by administering a treatment.

Caution is required with the use of other antiarrhythmic agents belonging to the same group.

Onset of a new arrhythmia

Ventricular tachycardia

Evidence based on the timing

The event is more likely to be explained by a proarrhythmic drug effect when the arrhythmia appears within hours or days after the beginning of treatment or a dosage increase.

Class Ic antiarrhythmic agents appear to be closely implicated in the occurrence of this severe adverse reaction (as well as in the aggravation of a pre-existing ventricular tachycardia).

Clinical evidence

This is based on the existence of risk factors.

Of course, this evidence is also valid when a ventricular tachycardia (with the same morphology) is aggravated by an antiarrhythmic treatment.

- Established risk factors
  - history of sustained ventricular tachycardia or ventricular fibrillation
  - underlying heart disease and/or altered left ejection fraction
  - heart failure
  - diuretic and/or digitalis treatment.
- Controversial risk factors
  - dosage of antiarrhythmic drug

However, it has been established that when the patient has a history of sustained ventricular tachycardia or ventricular fibrillation, class Ic antiarrhythmic agents in high doses are a significant risk factor for a proarrhythmic effect.

— aggravation of arrhythmia with physical effort.

Few studies have considered this problem. However, the widening of the sinusal QRS complexes with physical effort could be an important risk factor with class Ic antiarrhythmic drugs.

Torsades de pointes

Evidence based on the timing
- Any time to onset is compatible.
- The course on discontinuation of the treatment, and in particular the evolution of repolarization (normalization of QT interval), is decisive evidence (even though corrective treatments are often instituted).

Torsades de pointes associated with antiarrhythmics are not necessarily dose-dependent. Idiosyncratic phenomena can even occur (quinidine).

Clinical evidence
Here, too, identifying the (classic) factors that promote the occurrence of torsades de pointes is an important step:

- hypokalemia, to which a diuretic or laxative treatment often contributes
- hypomagnesemia
- bradycardia
- sex (female preponderance) and/or old age.

Note that the drug-induced causes of torsades de pointes are not limited to antiarrhythmic agents and that the following may also be responsible:

- *psychotropic agents (antipsychotics and antidepressants)*
- *vasodilatators*
- *antibacterials (erythromycin, etc.);*
- *H_1-receptor antagonists (terfenadine, astemizole).*

Management

This is primarily preventive

- Avoid any unjustified antiarrhythmic treatment.
- Any antiarrhythmic prescription should be preceded by an evaluation of renal and hepatic functions as well as by a search for—and if necessary correction of—hypokalemia.

- All antiarrhythmic treatments need
  to be monitored:

  - clinically
  - by electrocardiographic
    assessments. In most cases,
    prolonged Holter monitoring is
    essential
  - by laboratory tests (serum or
    plasma potassium level).

Occurrence of a proarrhythmic effect

- If the proarrhythmic effect seems
  minor:
  - stop the treatment immediately
  - reconsider the appropriateness of
    the treatment
  - if renewed treatment appears
    unavoidable, the dosage should be
    prudent, accompanied by
    extremely close monitoring.

- If the proarrhythmic effect is **severe**:
  - transfer the patient immediately
    to a cardiac care unit
  - emergency medical assistance may
    be necessary.

Severe proarrhythmic effects include:

- *Onset of runs of extrasystoles
  accompanied by functional signs
  (particularly faintness or syncope)
  and by hemodynamic changes.*

- *And/or severe ECG changes*
  - *onset of nonsustained
    ventricular tachycardia*
  - *ventricular tachycardia*

References

Bigger JT, Sahar DI. Clinical types of proarrhythmic response to antiarrhythmic drugs. Am J Cardiol 1987; 59: 2E–9E.

Jackman WM, Friday KJ, Anderson JL, Alliot EM. The long QT syndrome: a critical review, new clinical observations and a unifying hypothesis. Progr Cardiovasc Dis 1988; 31: 115–72.

Velebit V, Podrid P, Lown B, Cohen BH, Graboys TB. Aggravation and provocation of ventricular arrhythmics by antiarrhythmic drugs. Circulation 1982; 65: 886–94.

Conduction disorders

Catherine Chapelon

Sinoatrial, atrioventricular and intraventricular conduction disturbances are defined by their electrocardiographic features.

A recording in all leads is necessary.

Implicated drugs

- Antiarrhythmic agents
- Beta-blockers
- Calcium channel-blocking drugs (except for 1,4-dihydropyridines and diltiazem)
- Digitalis glycosides
- Anthracyclines

Management

This is the same as for arrhythmias. The treatment must be stopped, and the patient transferred to an intensive care unit if the conduction disturbance is severe and is symptomatic (second-degree and especially third-degree AV block).

Myocardial dysfunction
Catherine Chapelon

Medicines may induce ischemic heart disease, apart from any atheromatous lesion, via several mechanisms.

- Reduced coronary flow: hypotensives, negatively inotropic agents, vasodilators
- Induction of coronary spasm: ergot alkaloids, ergotamine, bromocriptine, ritodrine, terbutaline, certain prostaglandins
- Coronary "steal": calcium channel blockers
- Thrombosis: oral contraceptives (estrogens and progestins)

Other drug-induced cardiomyopathies are rare, whether they be related to toxicity (anticancer drugs), hypersensitivity (antibiotics) or metabolic disturbances (any agent capable of causing hypocalcemia).

Pericardial disease
Catherine Chapelon

All anticoagulant or antiplatelet drugs can cause hemopericarditis.

Other types of pericardial involvement are exceptional, except for drug-induced lupus (SLE).

Heart failure
Catherine Chapelon

Drugs can produce heart failure either directly by negative inotropism, or indirectly by salt and water retention.

Direct mechanism
Beta-blockers
Calcium channel blockers (particularly the nondehydropyridines)
Antiarrhythmic agents
Cyclophosphamide, anthracyclines, interferon

Indirect mechanism
Estrogens and progestins (oral contraceptives)
Androgens
Glucocorticoids
NSAIDs

12 Psychiatric disorders

Charles Peretti

Many drugs may induce psychiatric disorders which will vary considerably with the drug in question and the patient. Since drug-induced acute psychiatric states are eminently treatable by stopping the offending medicine, a drug-related origin must be considered in all such disorders.

Drug-induced confusional states

Definition

The clinical picture may combine:

- Temporospatial disorientation;

   The patient is disorientated in time and/or space. He goes to the wrong room, makes mistakes and his circadian rhythm changes.

- Disorders of higher cerebral functions: difficulty in focusing attention with distractibility, memory disturbances with complete amnesia (amnesic gap) for the confused period, which can provide a retrospective diagnosis;

   There is intellectual dullness, the patient being unable to understand questions, or do simple mental arithmetic.

- Behavioral disorders: mostly agitation, occasionally inhibition;

- Dream-like delirium

   The delirium, with added hallucinations, is experienced by the patient with intensity.

- Hallucinations;

   The patient suffers from predominantly visual hallucinations (scenes with action, mainly featuring animals).

Adverse Drug Reactions. A Practical Guide to Diagnosis and Management. Edited by C. Bénichou.
©1994 John Wiley & Sons Ltd.

- Mistaken identity;
- Mood swings;

Variability of the symptoms with time is characteristic of the confusional states;

The symptoms get worse in the evening, and there is daytime somnolence.

The **clinical course** is usually favorable if the offending medication is stopped, but the ultimate resolution depends on the general state of the patient. The amnesic gap persists.

Other clinical patterns

By symptom

- **Pure hallucinations**: the patient is completely involved with his dreams, with aggravation at night;
- **Antisocial behavior**: fugues, injury to self and others, criminal behavior;
- **Poor concentration**: fluctuating vigilance, variable attention, temporospatial disorientation;
- **In association with metabolic disorders**: hydroelectrolytic imbalance (dehydration, renal diabetes, etc.), which are often the consequences of the confusion.

Psychodysleptic drugs, anticholinergics, dopamine and its stimulants (e.g. amphetamines) can cause this type of disorder.

Anxiety and perplexity are common features of mental confusion.

By underlying pathology

- **Depression**;

There can be additional fits or cardiac dysrhythmias (tricyclic antidepressants).

- **Manic crises**;
- **Acute or chronic psychosis** with addition of psychosis-induced delirium to the mental confusion.

Prolonged pseudodementias are seen in the elderly.

By drug

- **Malignant neuroleptic syndrome**: consists of **confusion, rigidity,**

This reaction is unpredictable and nondose-dependent. Predisposing

autonomic nervous system dysfunction and **fever**.

factors can include dehydration and extreme fatigue. Neuroleptics must be stopped, the patient sent to an intensive care unit and dantrolene and/or bromocriptine used as necessary.

Signs of severity

- **Persistence of the confusion**: despite stopping the offending drug (and after its complete elimination), and correcting the electrolyte imbalance;

  Lack of improvement requires identification of irreversible organic damage or another cause for the confusional state. In the same way, drug-induced irreversible organic dysfunction may give rise to persistent metabolic disorders.

- **Impairment of consciousness** indicates a severe CNS disturbance.
- **Poor general condition: in the elderly** and patients with multisystem disease.

  Multiple organ failure such as heart failure, dysrhythmias, poor clotting function or renal disease with edema are factors aggravating the prognosis of the confusional state.

Identification of causes

Organic diseases

These are the major causes of confusional states and should be considered first. Any disease with potential impact on the CNS is a potential cause. A general check-up will identify nondrug etiologies:

- metabolic

  Hypo- or hyperglycemia, dehydration, water intoxication, hyperthyroidism.

- infectious

  Meningitis, encephalitis, septicemia, malaria, some viral infections.

- primary CNS disorders

  Hemorrhage, stroke, head injuries, brain tumor.

- secondary cerebral hypoxia

  Myocardial infarction, pulmonary embolus, severe anemia.

- most importantly, **nondrug intoxication**;

  Chronic or acute alcoholism.

- accidental and industrial intoxication.

  Carbon monoxide poisoning, mushrooms, lead, mercury, trichloroethylene, insecticides.

Evidence implicating a drug (see Table 1)

The essential argument is chronological; the symptoms should appear after the drug is started, especially if they appear within the first week of treatment. The lack of other causes is an indirect argument.

Sometimes the confusion is due to accumulation of drugs or the alteration of kinetics, for example lithium salts and renal failure, or association with antiinflammatories (NSAIDs, aspirin).

Table 1   Drugs implicated in confusional states. Incidence of side effects: + = low; + + = moderate; + + + = high

Psychotropic agents
    Amphetamines and anorectic derivatives +
    Barbiturates + + +
    Benzodiazepines + +
    Neuroleptics + +
    Lithium + +
    Antidepressants + + +
	Respiratory drugs
	    Theophylline + +

Antiparkinsonians
    L-dopa + +
    Amantadine + +
    Anticholinergics + + +
    Bromocriptine +
	Antibiotics
	    Penicillin G, cephalosporins +
	    Aminoglycosides +
	    Nalidixic acid +
	    Trimethoprim-sulfamethoxazole +

	Antituberculosis agents
	    Isoniazid +
	    Rifampicin +
	    Ethambutol +
	    Ethionamide +

Antihypertensive agents
    Alpha-methyldopa + +
    Prazosin +
    Beta-blockers +
	Antiviral agents
	    Acyclovir +

Anticholinergics + + +	**Antimalarials** Chloroquine +

Anticonvulsants + +	**Antifungal agents**
	    Griseofulvin + +
	    5-fluorocytosin and imidazole
	      derivatives + +

Analgesics Opioids + +	

NSAIDs
    Indomethacin +
	Hormones
	    ACTH, corticosteroids +
	    Thyroxine +

Cardiologic drugs
    Digitalis + +
    Antiarrhythmics +
    Diuretics +
	Miscellaneous
	    Baclofen + +
	    Ketamine + + +

Antihistamines
    Anti-H$_1$ +
    Anti-H$_2$ + + +	

In the introverted patient the diagnosis is **easily missed**, especially in the elderly. Any **sedative or hypnotic** drugs at high doses and given long term can cause confusion. **Benzodiazepines** are the most common drugs implicated at present, mainly because their use is so widespread. **Barbiturates** and **bromides**, both during treatment and after abrupt stoppage, may give the same problems.

Tricyclic antidepressants and **MAOIs** with anticholinergic properties can cause confusion in the elderly who are very susceptible. The confusion is in line with age and high blood levels, and other side effects such as blurred vision and urinary retention may be missing.

Amitryptiline and imipramine are the most frequent drugs involved in this category. Neuroleptics are implicated by their anticholinergic properties.

Management

If no organic cause is found for the confusion, all non life-saving drugs should be stopped. It may be difficult to decide which drug was responsible if several drugs were taken or if there is also an element of organ failure. If in doubt, all medications should be stopped except those absolutely necessary.

IV physostigmine in the treatment of anticholinergic syndrome is not advisable because of the undesirable cardiac side effects.

Agitation

Definition

Agitation is defined as a state of motor hyperactivity of variable intensity from permanently awake to a clastic crisis. Verbal communication may be increased, normal or totally abolished.

Clinical variations

Anxiety may be associated.

Additional central signs of anxiety such as worry, apprehension, fear, fright, panic.

An **epileptic fit**, sometimes without a past history, may occur.

A CNS disorder should be borne in mind.

Agitation can be seen in other psychiatric disorders: manic crisis in the psychotic patient with delirium (acute manic attack, schizophrenia), confusion (see previous section).

Signs of severity

A major state of agitation with clastic or epileptic fury may be life-threatening for the patient or lead to criminal behavior.

Etiology and evidence implicating a drug

A primary psychiatric cause should be thought of first, bearing in mind the possibility of a drug reaction in a known psychiatric patient. A short time to onset is in favor of a drug-related origin; i.e. the crisis occurs within a few days or even a few hours after starting the drug. Amphetamines and antidepressants are most often involved. Benzodiazepine or barbiturate withdrawal, following abrupt stoppage, are another possibility.

Mental inhibition

Definition

The inhibition is also motor with general slowing down, and may reach a stuporous state with a completely mute patient.

Clinical variations

Purely motor inhibition may be due to a neuroleptic syndrome, with relative preservation of speech, extrapyramidal syndrome (cogwheel sign and parkinsonian-type tremor).

Anxiety associated with the inhibition is relatively common, and is seen in depression with psychological inhibition.

Signs of severity

A patient who refuses to eat and is completely mute requires urgent treatment.

Etiology and evidence implicating a drug

A psychiatric disorder comes to mind first, but this does not exclude a drug reaction as a trigger.

Some antidepressants have a stimulant effect, but somnolence can appear in some patients. Drowsiness is also a frequent side effect of the neuroleptics such as chlorpromazine, thioridazine and some sedative phenothiazines (levomepromazine, etc.). The initial drowsiness wears off spontaneously, but oversedation persists in some patients. Neuroleptics can cause akinesia.

Antihypertensive drugs (e.g. methyldopa, clonidine) can often cause fatigue, lethargy and drowsiness. Indoramin and prazosin can also cause drowsiness and slowing down.

Beta-blocking drugs have been said to cause a feeling of lethargy following physical activity. This could be due to a low cardiac output.

Mood changes: depression and mania

Affective disorders can be put into two major groups: depression and mania.

Dysphoria is due to a modification of the equilibrium of emotions giving a feeling of abnormal and variable affect of a different quality and tone to the normal mood.

Emotional indifference or schizoid states are also affective disorders but are seen in psychotic disorders (acute delusional state, schizophrenia, etc.).

Dysphoria can be assessed by comparison with the previous emotional state (considered normal) of the patient.

Depression

Definition

Depression is characterized by mental pain, psychomotor atonia and somatic signs of depression.

The mental pain causes sadness, self-accusation, tears, self-depreciation, a global pessimism and suicidal thoughts.

The depressive syndrome is of variable severity; suicidal thoughts are the markers of severe depression.

Psychomotor atonia includes motor inhibition, slow and rare speech, lack of facial expression, slow and rare movements, slowness of thought, apragmatism, asthenia and slow intestinal transit. Somatic signs of depression include insomnia, anorexia, weight loss, amenorrhea, and loss of libido.

Clinical variations

Severe forms: melancholic states

Major atonia, sad delirious thoughts, major suicide risk, rapid global motor inhibition, almost complete insomnia.

Slight forms

Some atonia or slight fatigue, insomnia and anxiety, sadness.

Pseudodementia

In the elderly, sometimes confused with mental deterioration or dementia.

One major symptom

Severe insomnia, sudden anxiety attacks
or severe prolonged fatigue.

Etiology and evidence implicating a drug (see Table 2)

It may be difficult to differentiate
primary depression from drug-induced
apathy, a toxic lethargic state due to
disease or drugs, or a reactive
depression caused by personal
circumstances.

*Neuroleptics have been accused of
causing depression, particularly in the
long-term treatment of schizophrenia,
but absolute proof of this has not
been established. Neuroleptics may
cause a pseudodepression because of
the induced psychomotor atonia.*

Tetrabenazine (a rauwolfia derivative) is
sometimes used in tardive dyskinesia,
and can in itself cause inhibition and
akinesia akin to depression.

*Propranolol, other beta-blockers and
disulfiram could also be responsible
for some depression, but there is no
conclusive evidence.*

Table 2 Drugs implicated in depression. Incidence of side effects: + = low;
+ + = moderate; + + + = high

Psychotropic agents Amphetamines and anorectic derivatives + + + Neuroleptics + +	Respiratory drugs Theophylline +
Antiparkinsonians L-dopa + +	Antituberculosis agents Ethionamide + +
Antihypertensive agents Reserpinics + + + Alpha-methyldopa + + Clonidine and similar + + + Prazosin + Beta-blockers +	Antimalarials Chloroquine + Antifungal agents Griseofulvin + + 5-fluorocytosin and imidazole derivatives + +
Analgesics Opioids +	Hormones ACTH, corticosteroids + + +
NSAIDs Indomethacin +	Miscellaneous Baclofen + + Disulfiram +
Antihistamines Anti-H2 + +	

When weaning from appetite-suppressant drugs such as amphetamines and fenfluramine a temporary depression can occur. This is also true for benzodiazepines.

Clinical course and management

The disorder can regress when the drug is stopped, but can also evolve on its own account, needing in that case the same therapeutic approach as a spontaneously arising illness.

Mania

Definition

The symptoms are the mirror image of those of depression, with mental and motor hyperactivity, rapidity of thought, distractibility, sleep disturbance, cheery mood and disturbed behavior featuring overspending, grandiose projects and megalomania.

There is also excessive familiarity and flight of ideas. The patient becomes increasingly agitated and exhausted, and there is a serious risk of dehydration and physical deterioration. In a few days, the patient becomes totally exhausted and wasted.

Clinical variations

Mild forms

Hypomania presents a patient full of zest and cheeriness, sometimes with sleep disturbance.

Severe forms

With delirious thoughts, and uncontrollable agitation. The patient can become violent. The severe manias are more commonly seen in patients with a history of bipolar disorder.

Etiology and evidence implicating a drug (see Table 3)

As with depressive illness, the diagnosis should eliminate the decompensation of a previous mania, some cerebral disorders or endocrine abnormalities.

Amphetamines can cause excitation and euphoria, but they are more often the cause of paranoid psychosis.

Table 3 Drugs implicated in manic states. Incidence of side effects: + =low; + + =moderate; + + + =high

Psychotropic agents	Antituberculosis agents
Amphetamines and anorectic derivatives + +	Isoniazid + + +
Antidepressants + + +	Ethionamide + +
	Hormones
Antiparkinsonians	ACTH, corticosteroids + + +
L-dopa +	
Amantadine +	Miscellaneous
Bromocriptine +	Disulfiram +

Thymoanaleptic drugs can switch the mood round, inducing a manic episode.

Drugs with anticholinergic properties used in Parkinson's disease can induce excitation and euphoria, often in association with alcohol intake.

The same effect can be seen when a healthy patient is abusing medicines, and in some schizophrenics.

Antidepressants are the most frequent drugs causing mania and hypomania; the symptoms may appear even in the first week of treatment.

Clinical course and management

The disorder can regress when the drug is stopped, but can also evolve on its own account, needing in that case the same therapeutic approach as a spontaneously arising illness.

Sleep disorders

Definition

Sleep disorders are defined as an alteration in the duration or the quality of sleep. The two types are insomnia and hypersomnia.

Insomnia has three subtypes: delayed sleep, broken sleep or early waking.

Signs of severity

Insomnia is severe if there is no sleep, or if there is associated confusion, agitation or psychotic symptoms (delusional ideas, hallucinations).

Etiology and evidence implicating a drug

Propranolol is occasionally responsible for some types of insomnia, oneirism and nightmares. Reserpine derivatives, pargyline, methyldopa and clonidine can cause similar problems.

Amphetamines cause insomnia, sometimes severe.

Antidepressants can cause sleep disorders.

Other drugs are well known for their excitatory effects: corticosteroids, thyroid hormones. Benzodiazepine withdrawal should be considered.

The commonest cause of hypersomnia is self-medication (hypnotic drugs, neuroleptics).

Eating disorders

Amphetamines and their derivatives are well known for their anorectic effect. Fluoxetine can also cause weight loss. All anticholinergic agents dry the mucosa and induce a dry mouth with glossitis or stomatitis and temporary anorexia.

The regression of anorexia during antidepressant therapy is not only due to the lift in mood, but rather to a specific effect of the drug on eating behavior.

Antidepressants and neuroleptics commonly cause weight gain, which can explain the patient's reluctance to take them.

Memory defects: amnesias

Definition

There is a distinction between:

- impairment of recent memory (anterograde amnesia), with intact memory for older events;
- retroactive amnesia or retrograde amnesia, with impaired memory for older events;
- anteroretrograde amnesia, which involves both.

Reversible memory defects have been seen in elderly (nondemented) patients with anticholinergic agents for Parkinson's disease, as well as in young chronic schizophrenia sufferers. Benzodiazepines have an anterograde amnesic effect taken advantage of by anesthesiologists.

Memory defects induced by long-term benzodiazepine therapy diminish with time because of tolerance.

Cognitive changes

The inability to focus attention can be caused by benzodiazepines, neuroleptics, some antidepressants and scopolamine.

Cognitive changes such as a reduced ability to concentrate and temporary amnesia have been suffered by patients taking methyldopa; such patients usually have an occupation requiring a persistent high degree of mental ability.

Some patients taking psychotropic agents complain of a subjective impairment of cognitive ability with mental fatigue and lethargy, which they find difficult to define, and which is mistaken for depression.

Some psychotropic drugs slow down reaction time (neuroleptics, benzodiazepines, sedative antidepressants).

Psychoses

Definition

The patient loses contact with reality, with delusions and/or hallucinations and/or disturbance in thinking (discordance, dissociation in thought processing) resulting in abnormally vague, unstructured and flowing speech.

Clinical variations

Psychoses can be acute or chronic. The former will be described as they are more often part of drug-induced syndromes.

In the better known acute delirium, some or all the elements described in the above definition may be present. The characteristic is the clinical variety and variation in time.

Paranoid delirium are more often present with predisposing personalities.

No drug has so far been implicated in the etiology of chronic psychoses. Some agents which are used in long-term therapy or are abused (LSD, cocaine, heroin, amphetamines, etc.) are responsible for medium-term psychotic symptoms.

Acute psychosis mimicking acute depression can appear spontaneously at adolescence or during an acute anxiety attack.

Signs of severity

These are: sudden attacks involving frequent impulsive actions, intense delusions or anxiety and frequent hallucinations, with the risk of injury to self and others.

Etiology and evidence implicating a drug (see Tables 4 and 5)

There may always be an underlying psychosis. Suspected agents would have been started in the previous three months. Pre-existing psychotic illness in the patient or his family

Table 4 Drugs implicated in psychoses. Incidence of side effects: + = low; + + = moderate; + + + = high

Psychotropic agents
    Amphetamines and anorectic derivatives + + +
    Antidepressants +
	Cardiologic drugs
	    Digitalis +

Antiparkinsonians
    L-dopa +
    Amantadine +
    Anticholinergics +
    Bromocriptine +
	Respiratory drugs
	    Ephedrine + + +
	Antituberculosis agents
	    Isoniazid + +

Antihypertensive agents
    Beta-blockers +
	Antimalarials
	    Chloroquine +

Anticholinergics +	Hormones ACTH, corticosteroids +

NSAIDs
    Indomethacin +
	Miscellaneous
	    Disulfiram + +

Table 5 Drugs implicated in hallucinations. Incidence of side effects: + = low; + + = moderate; + + + = high

Antiparkinsonians
    L-dopa + + +
    Amantadine + + +
    Anticholinergics + + +
    Bromocriptine + + +
	Antihistamines
	    Anti-H$_1$ + +
	    Anti-H$_2$ + +

Antihypertensive agents
    Clonidine and similar +
    Prazosin +
    Beta-blockers +
	Respiratory drugs
	    Ephedrine + + +
	    Beta-agonists: salbutamol + +

Anticholinergics + + +	Antiviral agents Acyclovir +

Analgesics
    Opioids + +
	Antimalarials
	    Chloroquine +

NSAIDs
    Indomethacin +
	Antifungal agents
	    5-fluorocytosin and imidazole derivatives +

Cardiologic drugs
    Digitalis + +
	Miscellaneous
	    Baclofen +
	    Ketamine + + +

increases the risk of psychotic reactions to drug therapy. Lipophilic beta-blocking agents such as propranolol can cause hallucinations, most often with alcoholics. Propranolol can also cause psychotic symptoms with increased dosage.

Antidepressants can cause or exacerbate hallucinations, and may unmask the delusions of a psychotic patient who could not express them previously.

Withdrawal syndromes

Drug withdrawal psychosis

The sudden cessation of treatment by patient or doctor in patients receiving long-term therapy with neuroleptics or antidepressants can cause acute psychotic manifestations.

Schizophrenia has been described in patients who stopped receiving neuroleptics for a different indication (e.g. for mania in a manic-depressive patient).

Some authors have a theory of "hypersensitivity psychosis" in patients for whom neuroleptics have been gradually stopped after long-term therapy, much in the same way as these patients seem to have hypersensitive dopaminergic receptors when they suffer from tardive dyskinesia. This effect on the mind could result in a psychosis.

Benzodiazepine and barbiturate withdrawal

The symptoms appear if the drug is stopped abruptly. There is rebound anxiety, insomnia, instability, agitation, even epileptic fits. Some modification of sensory perceptions is part of the syndrome, such as noise and light intolerance, and a subjective feeling of instability.

With barbiturates, insomnia may be associated with the rapid onset of epileptic fits and agitation. The drug should be restarted and a more gradual process of reduction in dosage established.

Clonidine

The rapid stoppage of clonidine therapy may cause agitation, insomnia, headaches, nausea, abdominal pain and hypertensive crisis.

Caffeine

Caffeine withdrawal can cause psychomotor inhibition and reduces mental capacity.

Table 6 gives a list of drugs implicated in withdrawal syndromes.

Table 6 Drugs implicated in withdrawal syndromes. Incidence of side effects: + = low; + + = moderate; + + + = high.

Psychotropic agents	Analgesics
Amphetamines and anorectic derivatives + + +	Opioids + + +
Barbiturates + + +	
Benzodiazepines + +	Respiratory drugs
	Ephedrine +
Antiparkinsonians	
L-dopa +	Miscellaneous
	Baclofen + + +
Antihypertensive agents	
Clonidine and similar + +	

13 Cytotoxic chemotherapy induced disorders

Philippe Solal-Céligny

Hyperpyrexia

The onset of fever in a patient receiving cytotoxic chemotherapy prompts the question of its origin: an infection, a fever related to the tumor itself, a drug-induced or other iatrogenic cause of fever.

Steroids and nonspecific antipyretics should never be started before a diagnosis is established.

An infectious cause is the first possibility to consider

Immediate full blood count

If the neutrophil count is below 1000/μL, an infectious complication is highly probable. Management includes:

- multiple cultures: blood, urine, skin lesions
- initiation of treatment with broad-spectrum antibiotics before the results of these tests are known.

If the neutrophil count is above 1000/μL, the usual diagnostic work-up for a pyrexia of unknown origin should be followed.

Look for a focus of infection and carry out swab and other cultures depending on the clinical picture

- throat
- lungs
- urinary tract
- IV catheter sites

Adverse Drug Reactions. A Practical Guide to Diagnosis and Management. Edited by C. Bénichou.
©1994 John Wiley & Sons Ltd.

Start antibiotics immediately in the following circumstances:

- depression of the immune response (hemopathy, multiple previous chemotherapies, weight loss)
- moderate neutropenia or lymphopenia
- use of IV infusion implants (catheters, etc.)
- possible tumor-related infection: bronchus, ENT, uterus.

A neoplastic cause ("specific" fever) should be sought, particularly in the following circumstances

- tumor not controlled by chemotherapy
  - clinical or radiographic changes
  - increased serum tumor markers
  - new tumor development associated with the pyrexia
- persistent pyrexia that is well tolerated
- no neutropenia or inflammatory reaction, and/or raised blood LDH
- lack of response to antibiotics
- transient but definite response to a low-dose NSAID (e.g. naproxen 125 mg orally).

Other causes of pyrexia are rare

Drugs

- hormones (e.g. high-dose progestogens)
- some cytotoxic drugs (hypersensitivity reaction)
  - *asparaginase*
  - *procarbazine*
  - *taxol*
  - *bleomycin*
  - *methotrexate*
  - *interleukin 2*
  - *interferons*

Other (nondrug) causes

- *venous thrombosis*
  - *lower limbs*
  - *pelvis*
  - *IV catheter site*
- *phlebitis or lymphangitis due to the sclerosing effect of drugs*
- *hemolytic anemia*

Neutropenia

Neutropenia is a very common complication of cancer chemotherapy due to the toxicity of these drugs on the granulocyte precursor cells in the bone marrow, which have a rapid rate of renewal.

The **degree** of neutropenia is determined by the nadir (lowest number of observed neutrophils granulocytes), which depends on:

- drugs used for chemotherapy
- *type (see Table 1)*
- *dose*
- *mode of administration*
- *delay between courses*

Table 1 Principal cytotoxic drugs affecting bone marrow

Drug family	Severe	Moderate	Minor or absent
Alkylating agents	caryolysin melphalan chlorambucil cyclophosphamide ifosfamide busulfan*		
Podophyllotoxins	etoposide (VP 16)	teniposide (VM 26)	
Vinca-alkaloids	vinorelbine	vindesine vinblastine	vincristine
Nitrosoureas	carmustine* & *** lomustine* & *** fotemustine* & ***		
Antimetabolites	cytarabine methotrexate** mercaptopurine hydroxyurea	5-fluorouracil fludarabine 2 chlor desoxyadenosine	
Anthracyclines and analogues	adriamycin epirubicin pirarubicin idarubicin mitoxantrone		
Antibiotics		mitomycin	bleomycin
Platins	carboplatin***	cisplatin	
Miscellaneous	dacarbazine	procarbazine alpha-interferon interleukin 2	asparaginase

*Delayed toxicity, nadir 3 to 5 weeks post-treatment.
**Possibly reversible with folinic acid.
***Toxicity mainly involving platelets.

- previous treatments
  - *radiotherapy affecting hematopoietic bone marrow*
  - *cumulative dose of previous courses of chemotherapy*
- age of patient
  - *higher incidence in older patients*
- stage of the neoplasm.
  - *tumor mass*
  - *bone marrow infiltration*

The **severity** of a neutropenia depends on:

- its **degree**
  - *nadir less than 1000 or 500/µL*
- its **duration**
  - *the number of days that the neutrophil granulocyte count is <500/µL*
- presence of factors increasing the likelihood of **infection**.
  - *poor performance status*
  - *potential sources of bronchial, urinary or venous infections*

The **time of onset** depends on:

- neutrophil granulocyte count immediately before initiating the treatment
  - *The interval is usually short: nadir 7–14 days after the first day of the cycle*
- drugs used.
  - *It is sometimes delayed (21–35 days): see Table 1*

Regular monitoring of **blood counts** are generally not of value because:

- they can be unnecessarily worrying: neutropenia is very common and not necessarily a complication;
- they can be falsely reassuring: a drop in neutrophil count can be very rapid.

Indications for a blood cell count are independent of the time and values of the previous test in the case of:

- fever
- septic shock, circulatory collapse, sudden deterioration of health, hypothermia;
- infection: tonsillitis (+ + +) or stomatitis, cystitis, bronchopneumonia.

Management depends on several factors.

- Admission to a **specialist hospital unit** is mandatory for febrile patients with a neutrophil count <500/µL.
- If the count is higher, hospital admission depends on:
  - clinical status of the patient: degree of fever, shivers, performance status
  - severity of neutropenia
  - likely natural course of the neutropenia (increasing or decreasing count), as suggested by the time and dose of the last cycle of chemotherapy.

Management of a severe ($< 500/\mu$L) febrile neutropenia

Initial investigations include: immediate blood cultures, chest radiography, urine culture and culture swabs from any site of infection.

Treatment should be initiated immediately (within 2 hours):

- antibiotics

- if necessary, hematopoietic growth factors: G-CSF or GM-CSF.

- *broad-spectrum drugs, IV rather than oral*

- *These drugs can also be administered prophylactically for the subsequent cycles of chemotherapy.*

Thrombocytopenia

This complication is less common than neutropenia, less predictable and difficult to treat.

The **severity** (i.e. the nadir) depends on:

- the chemotherapy drugs
  - *type (see Table 1)*
  - *dose*
  - *time interval between courses*
- previous treatments
- extent of the disease.

The **importance** depends on:

- primarily the severity
- presence of a potentially hemorrhagic lesion:
  - intestinal tumor
  - peptic ulcer
  - brain tumor.

A positive diagnosis of drug-induced thrombocytopenia can be made after excluding:

- disseminated intravascular coagulation (DIC), as assessed from blood levels of fibrinogen, fibrin degradation products (FDP), and soluble complexes
- thrombotic microangiopathy: hemolytic schistocytic anemia
- massive bone marrow metastases: erythromyelemia
- autoimmune paraneoplastic thrombocytopenia or latent thrombocytopenia as revealed by biological response modifier (alpha-interferon, interleukin 2).

Clinical evaluation includes a search for an occult hemorrhage, in particular of the retina.

The **treatment** combines:

- sometimes low-dose corticosteroids to reduce the risk of hemorrhage;
- platelet replacement, depending on:
  - *degree of thrombocytopenia*
  - *relative risk of hemorrhage*
  - *expected duration*
  - *risk of alloimmunization*

Anemia

Anemia is frequently associated with cancer and is often caused by a number of factors:

- deficiencies in iron or folates
- acute phase reaction
- chronic or subacute hemorrhage
- bone marrow infiltration
- direct toxicity due to chemotherapy and radiotherapy
- less often, microangiopathy-induced hemolysis.

Moreover, anemia may be masked by an associated hemoconcentration due to:

- intestinal fluid losses
- cisplatin therapy, producing extracellular hypovolemia.

There are potentially several mechanisms of chemotherapy-induced anemia:

- toxicity on the hematopoietic cell precursors;

- microangiopathy:
  - *mitomycin C (+ + +)*
  - *vinca-alkaloids*
  - *cyclophosphamide*
  - *cisplatinum*

- deficiencies, especially folic acid:
  - *methotrexate*

- myelodysplastic syndrome:
  - *after long-standing chemotherapy with specific drugs (alkylating agents)*
  - *and/or in certain types of cancers (multiple myeloma)*

The mechanism of the patient's anemia should be elucidated before any treatment is recommended, in particular before blood transfusion:

- reticulocyte count
- presence of schistocytes
- tests for acute phase reactants
- hemolysis: free bilirubin, haptoglobin
- if necessary, measurements of plasma and red cell volumes.

Coagulation defects

Some cytotoxic agents may cause serious disturbances in hemostasis and coagulation mechanisms:

- mithramycin

- asparaginase

- *thrombocytopenia*
- *thrombopathy*

- *fibrinopenia*
- *antithrombin-3 deficit, with an increased risk of thrombosis*
- *increase in prothrombin time*

Gastrointestinal disorders

Cytotoxic-induced gastrointestinal disorders are:

- frequent
- sometimes severe, giving rise to disorders such as renal failure, dehydration, hyperkalemia, alkalosis or rapid weight loss
- often the cause of the patient's reluctance to begin or continue a course of chemotherapy.

However, these disorders can be prevented or easily treated in the vast majority of cases.

Nausea/vomiting

Symptoms are due to the action of the drugs on the chemoreceptor trigger zone located at the base of the fourth ventricle.

There are several categories of disorders (see Table 2):

Table 2   Emetic potential of cytotoxic agents

Highly emetic	Moderately emetic	Mildly emetic
Cisplatin	Actinomycin-D	Vincristine
Dacarbazine	Carboplatin	Vindesine
Mechlorethamine	Carmustine	Vinorelbine
Streptozotocin	Cyclophosphamide	Vinblastine
Melphalan (high dose)	Daunorubicin	Fludarabine
Taxol	Doxorubicin	Bleomycin
	Epirubicin	
	Ifosfamide	
	Methotrexate	
	Procarbazine	
	Cytarabine	

1. Nausea/vomiting preceding the chemotherapy, of a clearly psychogenic etiology

Management:

- *additional information on the likely effects of chemotherapy*
- *relaxation therapy*
- *anxiolytic treatment*

2. Nausea/vomiting within 24 hours of the start of chemotherapy

Symptom intensity depends on

- type of drug
- dose

- patient's personality

- the mode of drug administration: environment, rate of infusion, etc.

- *slightly more frequent in women*
- *reduced incidence and intensity with tobacco and alcohol abuse.*

Nausea/vomiting may have **adverse consequences**:

- peptic gastroesophagitis (Mallory-Weiss syndrome);
- inability to take drugs orally;
- dehydration, metabolic alkalosis, hypokalemia and renal insufficiency (with increased toxicity of some agents);
- refusal of the patient to continue treatment.

Treatment should be **prophylactic** because:

- it is easier than curative
- there is a carry-on phenomenon with a risk of recurrence.

There are many effective drugs (see Table 3). The choice depends on:

- *type of chemotherapy*
- *risk of adverse effect varying from patient to patient (e.g. extrapyramidal syndrome with dopamine antagonists more frequent in young patients)*
- *cost of treatment.*

Combinations must avoid drugs:

- *with the same mode of action*
- *with similar side effects.*

3. "Late" nausea/vomiting

This persists for more than 24–48 hours after stopping cytotoxic therapy.

Before attributing the symptoms to the cancer chemotherapy, other causes should be excluded, especially if there has been a symptom-free interval between the end of the course of chemotherapy and the reoccurrence of nausea/vomiting

Table 3 Main prophylactic and curative drugs used to treat cytotoxic drug-induced nausea/vomiting*

Mechanisms of action	DCI	Administration	Adult dosage	Side-effects
Dopamine antagonists	metoclopramide	oral (tablet, syrup) inj. IV, IM	10 to 60 mg/day	somnolence extrapyramidal syndrome
Serotonin antagonists	ondansetron	oral, IV	8 to 32 mg/day	headaches constipation
	granisetron	IV	3 mg/day	headaches constipation
Corticosteroids	methyl-prednisolone	IV	60 to 240 mg/day	shock salt retention
	tetracosactide	IM, IV	1 mg	shock
Neuroleptics	chlorpromazine	oral, IM, IV	25 to 150 mg/day	somnolence extrapyramidal syndrome orthostatic hypotension

*Other pharmaceutical (anxiolytics) or non-pharmaceutical treatments can be used in association.

More specifically, these have to be ruled out:

- *hypercalcemia*
- *bowel obstruction*
- *raised intracranial pressure*
- *renal failure*
- *hepatic disorder: tumor-, virus- or drug-induced*
- *hyponatremia (Schwartz-Bartter syndrome)*

The treatment of late nausea/vomiting is difficult:

- The efficacy of standard antiemetics (dopamine or serotonin inhibitors) is limited.
- Psychological factors play an important role.
- Benzodiazepines and low-dose neuroleptics appear to be the most effective agents.
- Effective prevention of immediate nausea/vomiting (i.e. occurring within 24 hours of starting chemotherapy) avoids the occurrence of late nausea/vomiting.

Diarrhea

Diarrhea is a rare complication of cytotoxic chemotherapy. It is important to exclude a "false diarrhea."

There are several complications of
diarrhea:

- *metabolic changes*
- *rapid weight loss*
- *dehydration and renal insufficiency*

Diarrhea is often associated with mucositis and, especially, stomatitis. The most frequently involved drugs are 5-fluorouracil, cytosine arabinoside and methyl glyoxal.

Constipation

All vinca alkaloids—especially vincristine—can cause a paralytic ileus that:

- occurs within 3–7 days of treatment
- is severe enough to mimic a surgical obstruction
- responds well to cautious doses of prostigmine.

Constipation is also a complication of antiserotonin antiemetics. There may be synergy with vinca alkaloids on gastrointestinal motility.

Stomatitis

Definition

This category includes all drug-induced disorders of the buccal cavity, which have multiple and often complex mechanisms:

- direct mucosal toxicity of some cytotoxic agents
- local or regional dental infections and periodontitis
- less often, thrombocytopenia-induced buccal hemorrhages
- salivary disorders, particularly after radiotherapy.

Stomatitis can be a **serious condition**:

- It may be the initial focus of a disseminated infection.
- It may not allow the patient to eat normally, resulting in rapid and massive weight loss.
- It may be extremely painful, leading to serious psychological consequences and poor patient compliance with treatment.

Mucosal toxicity

Mucositis is the result of any toxicity acting directly on the mucosa of the mouth and lips, that is renewed every 5–15 days.

The causative drugs are primarily those acting specifically on the cycle:

- *5-fluorouracil*
- *methotrexate*
- *actinomycin D*
- *adriamycin*
- *cyclophosphamide*
- *bleomycin*
- *etoposide*

Mucositis usually occurs 7–14 days after a course of chemotherapy.

Clinical signs and symptoms occur progressively:

- *burning sensation of the mouth and tongue*
- *erythematous areas*
- *ovoid ulcerations with necrotic centers surrounded with erythema*

Without treatment, spontaneous healing takes 7–14 days.

The treatment can be:

- **preventive**
  - *good oral hygiene*
  - *sucking ice cubes during infusions of cytotoxic agents (5-FU)*
  - *sucralfate or allopurinol*

- **sometimes specific**
  - *folinic acid if methotrexate is implicated*

- **difficult when** the mucositis has already become **established.**
  - *avoid all irritant or acidic food*
  - *liquidized diet*
  - *mouthwash combining bicarbonate, local anesthetic, diluted antiseptics*
  - *anesthetic gel applied before meals*

If the dose is not lowered, there is relapse of the mucositis with every course of chemotherapy

Focal regional infections

The following may be affected:

- The oral cavity, especially subsequent to mucositis
- the teeth (pulp) or periodontal area.

Oral infections

The main infective agents are:

- *gram-negative bacilli (*E. coli, Pseudomonas*)*
- Staphylococcus aureus
- *fungi:* Candida *(+ + +),* Torulopsis
- *viruses: herpes simplex (+ + +),* CMV

The treatment can be:

- **preventive**
  - *good oral and dental hygiene:*
    - *prophylactic extractions of affected teeth before chemotherapy*
    - *removal of ill-fitting dental prostheses*
    - *prophylactic treatment of pre-existing infections: pulpitis, gingivitis, periodontitis*

- mouthwash comprising 0.1% chlorhexidine
- possibly prophylactic antifungal treatment

- **curative**, after onset, depending on the causal agent diagnosed clinically or by culture.

- *clinically: thrush, labial herpes, etc.*
- *microbiologically: oral swabs, but polymicrobial infections are a common finding.*

Dental infections

Undetected and frequent before starting treatment, they expose the patient to several risks:

They are located:

- *in one or several teeth: pulpitis*
- *around the tooth: periapical infection, periodontitis, gingivitis.*

- They may extend during treatment to involve the gums or jaw bone.

- They may serve as an initial focus of an oral infection, and of bacteremia with secondary localizations, for example on a central venous catheter.

The treatment is mainly **preventive**:

- *full clinical and radiological dental check-up before starting treatment*
- *if possible, conservative dental treatment*
- *if dental extractions are necessary, they should be carried out with antibiotic cover for at least 10 days before the neutrophil count drops below 500/µL*
- *gentle toothbrushing and use of mouthwashes during treatment*
- *as soon as possible, all nonurgent dental treatments should be completed before the next course of chemotherapy.*

Neurological disorders

Peripheral neuropathies

Peripheral neuropathy is a common complication of cytotoxic chemotherapy, and may lead to serious complications.

Other causes must be excluded before the diagnosis of drug-induced neuropathy is established:

- nerve root or trunk compression
- neoplastic meningitis
- postradiation myelitis
- paraneoplastic neuropathy
- neuropathy due to vitamin deficiency.

Table 4　Main cytotoxic drugs inducing peripheral neuropathy and the various clinical presentations

Drug	Specific features
Cisplatinum	• Very common after a cumulative dose of 600 mg/m^2, but reactions are possible with lower doses, especially if high doses per course have been used. • Additional risk for alcoholic or female patients, and cotreatment with vinca-alkaloids. • Symptoms start in the lower limbs with subjective sensory disturbances, paresthesia, abolition of sense of vibration. • Even after stopping the drug, there is a risk of worsening, with additional motor symptoms, upper limb involvement and amyotrophy.
Carboplatin	• Similar to cisplatinum. Reactions rarely occur before a cumulative dose of $\leqslant$2500 mg/m^2. Probable synergistic toxicity with cisplatin, prohibiting any replacement of one with the other.
Vinca alkaloids (vincristine + + +)	• In the acute phase, especially after a high dose (vincristine >2 mg), there is a risk of paralytic ileus and urine retention. • With cumulative doses, signs of peripheral neuropathy with areflexia first, followed by motor symptoms and superficial sensory disturbances. • After stopping the drug, the symptoms do not worsen, but improve slowly although there are sequelae (permanent loss of tendon reflexes).
Alpha-interferon	• Rare sensorimotor peripheral neuropathies possibly potentiated by vinca alkaloids.
Taxol	• Reversible sensorimotor peripheral neuropathy; the risk is increased when high doses are used per course (>250 mg/m^2).

Table 4 lists the main cytotoxic drugs that induce peripheral neuropathy and its clinical presentation.

Central nervous system toxicity

Also called "toxic encephalopathies," these complications are:

- rare
- but many drugs have been implicated
- very severe, often lethal or having serious sequelae, especially in children.

Table 5 illustrates the main cytotoxic drugs implicated and the clinical presentations.

Table 5 Main cytotoxic drugs inducing toxic encephalopathy, and specific clinical features (with the exception of complications of intrathecal administration)

Drug	Clinical features
Methotrexate	• Only after high single doses (>500 mg/m^2). • Either acute reversible encephalopathy, with confusion, seizures and hemiparesis or, after repeated doses, chronic irreversible encephalopathy with dementia, motor deficit and cerebral atrophy. • Major potentiation with cerebral irradiation given before high-dose methotrexate.
Cytosine arabinoside	• Only following high intermittent doses (>500 mg/m^2), with an increased frequency depending on the total dose per course (very high incidence for doses >18 g/m^2), and in the elderly. • Symptoms mainly confined to the cerebellum (ataxia, dysmetria), followed by a possibility of coma, motor deficit. • Occasionally fatal, more often reversible and without sequelae.
5-Fluorouracil	• Acute, reversible, dose-dependent cerebellar disorders; higher risk with bolus administration, cotreatment with folinic acid, alpha-interferon and cisplatin. • Very rarely, chronic irreversible encephalopathy.
Ifosfamide	• Acute encephalopathy with somnolence, confusion, seizures and coma. • Mainly in children treated with high doses. • Usually reversible, but death may occur.
L-asparaginase	• Acute reversible encephalopathy. • Mainly in children, after a single high dose.
Fludarabine	• Chronic encephalopathy with cortical blindness, dementia, coma and tetraparesis. • Frequent after a single high dose, very rare after fractioning the dose over 4–5 days.
Interleukin 2	• Possible cerebral edema. • Very rare encephalopathies.

Urinary tract disorders
Renal failure and other renal disorders

Renal failure is a serious complication of cytotoxic chemotherapy because:

- it may be irreversible
- it increases the toxicity of other drugs
- it reduces the possibility of continuing with the full course of chemotherapy.

Before concluding that renal failure is due to drug toxicity, other causes should first be eliminated:

- mechanical obstruction of the ureter due to a tumor or postradiation retroperitoneal fibrosis
- massive cell destruction with hyperuricemic nephropathy (leukemias, lymphomas)
- paraneoplastic glomerulopathy.

Table 6 presents the characteristics of the main cytotoxic drugs that cause renal damage.

Cystitis

Cyclophosphamide and ifosfamide can lead to acute hemorrhagic cystitis with the additional risks of:

- in the short term, anemia, urethral obstruction with blood clots
- in the medium term, bladder sclerosis
- in the long term, secondary urothelial cancer

Acute cystitis may be prevented by:

- extensive diuresis
- previous and simultaneous administration of an uroprotective agent: mesna.

Table 6   Main cytotoxic agents inducing renal disorders

Drug	Specific features
Cisplatin	• Often preceded by electrolyte changes, hypomagnesemia, salt-depleting tubular disease (hypovolemia). • The renal impairment may be severe, often only partially reversible, and dose-dependent (with no cumulative toxicity). • This complication can be prevented by fractioning of the dose and, more importantly, preventive hyperhydration.
Methotrexate	• Renal failure can be induced by tubular precipitates only at high doses. • May be prevented by high-volume alkaline diuresis. • Renal failure can add substantially to the toxicity of the drug to bone marrow and mucous membranes
Mitomycin C	• Possible renal failure associated with a thrombotic microangiopathy.
Cyclo-phosphamide	• Rare syndrome of abnormal secretion of ADH.
Ifosfamide	• Possible proximal tubular disease (hypophosphoremia).
Streptozocin	• Possible subacute tubulointerstitial nephropathy (acidosis, hypokalemia).

Liver test abnormalities

Liver test abnormalities are frequent during anticancer therapy, and the causes are multiple and sometimes combined:

- specific liver damage, either multinodular metastases of a solid tumor, diffuse infiltration (hemopathy) or extrinsic neoplastic compression of the biliary tract.

  Liver injury is often cholestatic with or without jaundice. However, in the case of multiple metastases or massive infiltration, the injury can be hepatocellular and at times fulminant.

- Viral hepatitis, posttransfusional in particular, but also as a complication of immunodepression (CMV, herpes).
- Liver damage of ischemic origin (heart failure, constrictive pericarditis).
- Damage caused by external irradiation.
- Steatosis and/or cholestasis due to prolonged parenteral nutrition.
- Paraneoplastic syndrome, most often expressed as cholestasis.
- Toxicity of antineoplastics or supportive drugs such as antibiotics, antiemetics or analgesics. The principal anticancer drugs responsible for liver damage and their clinical characteristics are presented in Table 7.

Veno-occlusive disease of the liver is characterized by an obstruction of the central or sublobular veins by a loose connective tissue, causing congestion and necrosis of

Table 7   Principal antineoplastic drugs responsible for liver injury

Drug	Characteristics
Asparaginase	High frequency of hepatocellular hepatitis and/or acute hepatic failure (decrease in fibrinogen and antithrombin III).
Azathioprine	Cholestasis, infrequent.
Cytosine-Arabinoside	Hepatocellular hepatitis observed in 20% of cases at usual doses and up to 50% of cases at high doses.
Dacarbazine (DTIC)	Frequent (up to 50% of cases) and sometimes very serious injury. Often associated with eosinophila.
Floxuridine (FUdR)	Hepatocellular hepatitis or sclerosing cholangitis after perfusion of hepatic artery. Risk of acute cholecystitis (preventive cholecystectomy).
Interferon alpha	Rare hepatocellular hepatitis, probably due to exacerbation of pre-existing liver disease.
Mercaptopurine Tioguanine	After long term treatment (at least 2 months) hepatocellular or cholestatic hepatitis. Risk increased by doxorubicine?
Methotrexate	Chronic hepatitis and cirrhosis after prolonged administration at low doses.
Mithramycin	High frequency of acute hepatocellular hepatitis (>50% of cases).

Table 8 Antineoplastic drugs responsible for veno-occlusive disease of the liver

At usual doses	After preparation for bone marrow transplantation (high doses)
Azathioprine	Busulfan
Cytosine-arabinoside	Cyclophosphamide
Dacarbazine	BCNU (Carmustine) + etoposide?
Mercaptopurine	CCNU (Lomustine)
Thioguanine	Mitomycin

the corresponding hepatic territory. This liver disease is observed particularly during anticancer therapy, after chemotherapy at the usual doses or, above all, after preparation for bone marrow transplantation (13–20% of cases), combining chemotherapy at high doses and total body irradiation (Table 8). The hepatic injury is mainly hepatocellular and occurs within the month following preparation for the transplantation.

Respiratory disorders

Drug-induced lung disorders are:

- fairly frequent with some cytotoxic agents;
- severe, because in the acute phase they may induce adult respiratory distress syndrome (ARDS) and, in the longer term, permanent functional sequelae;
- difficult to diagnose, particularly with a chest infection and/or carcinomatosis (lymphangitis);
- typically presenting as an interstitial pneumonia.

Several factors are involved:

- direct cellular toxicity to the cells of the alveolocapillary membrane
- hypersensitivity reaction
- increased capillary permeability
- bronchial or bronchiolar edema, with stenosis.

Positive diagnosis

Symptoms are variable:

- abnormal chest x-ray during routine check-up
- subacute disease with fever, frequent dry cough, increasing dyspnea
- on occasions, rapid onset of ARDS.

Radiographic anomalies are nonspecific: interstitial infiltration, alveolar opacities mainly in the bases, lung contraction. Pleural effusions and mediastinal adenopathy are uncommon.

The **final diagnosis** in a patient treated with cytotoxic agents relies on several criteria, all of which are important:

1. The pathology being treated	- *higher incidence of drug-induced lung disorders in lymphomas* - *degree of immunosuppression* - *recent tumor progression*
2. Cardiovascular and respiratory history	- *chronic bronchitis* - *history of deep vein thrombosis* - *heart failure* - *cumulative dose of cardiotoxic drugs (anthracyclines)*
3. Most frequently involved drugs	*See Table 9*

Table 9 Cytotoxic drugs most frequently inducing respiratory disorders

Drugs	Characteristic features of respiratory disorder
Bleomycin	• Rarely, acute respiratory disorder due to hypersensitivity with fever, and steroid-sensitive eosinophilia. • More often, subacute fibrosis pneumonitis. • Exponential increase in risk with cumulative doses: low risk if <300 mg/m^2, higher risk with greater cumulative doses. • Potentiation of risk with additional thoracic radiotherapy, age >70, association with cisplatin, IV bolus injection. • Early detection, in some cases, by sequential measurements of alveolar carbon monoxide transfer. • Poor prognosis, fatal or with major sequelae. • Steroid therapy often prescribed without proven benefit.
Mitomycin C	• Rare, acute respiratory disorder, more often subacute fibrosing pneumonitis. • No threshold dose. • Same risk factors as with bleomycin. • Possible pulmonary edema due to increase in capillary permeability. • Frequent association with thrombotic microangiopathy.
Nitrosoureas (mainly BCNU)	• Clinical picture of ARDS, often serious, very often fatal. • Rare if the cumulative dose is <900 mg/m^2 of BNCU, higher risk with high single doses. • Smokers are more at risk.
Busulfan	• Most often after prolonged administration, at least 3 years. • Associated with hyperpigmentation and Addison-like syndrome. • A rapidly progressive fibrosis may perhaps be improved by corticosteroids.
Methotrexate	• Relatively frequent subacute symptoms such as cough, fever, dyspnea, eosinophilia, pumonary infiltrates and sometimes pleural reactions, or hyperacute onset. • No dose threshold. • Potentiated by underlying lymphomas, intermittent administration of bleomycin. • May be associated with pneumocystis pneumonia. • Sometimes with liver and renal toxicity. • Often reversible without sequelae, and there may be a more rapid recovery with steroids. • There may be no further reaction if methotrexate is used again (nevertheless, this is not recommended).
Cytarabine	• Pulmonary edema, onset 2 days to 3 weeks after the first dose. • Dose-related risk. • Favorable prognosis, with good response to high-dose steroids.
Procarbazine	• Rare, acute respiratory disorders, with good prognosis.
Vinca alkaloids (vindesine + + +)	• Rare, subacute respiratory disorders or pulmonary edema.
Interleukin 2	• Pulmonary edema, frequent episodes of pleurisy associated with high doses due to increased capillary permeability.

4. Hematological status
- *neutropenia and/or lymphopenia*
- *immediate post-aplasia phase (+ + +), period frequently associated with development of pulmonary infections*

5. Additional risk factors for drug-induced pneumopathies:
- *thoracic radiotherapy*
- *recent oxygen therapy*

6. Clinical, radiological, and biological features:
- *signs of heart failure*
- *other foci of infection*
- *specific radiological abnormalities (aspergilloma)*
- *eosinophilia*
- *increase in serum tumor markers*

7. Most importantly, endoscopic investigations:
- *Depending on the patient's cardiorespiratory status and his coagulation status:*

- in a specialized unit associated with microbiology laboratories able to give a rapid answer.
- *bronchial brushings*
- *bronchoalveolar lavage of the most affected areas with abnormal radiographic appearances*
- *biopsies of bronchial mucosa, endobronchial lesions and, possibly, transbronchial biopsies*
- *culture swabs for pyogenic bacteria, protozoa (Pneumocystis), fungal or viral infections*

8. Other microbiological and radiographic investigations:
- *cultures of blood and other body fluids*
- *test for microbial antigens*
- *serum antibody titres*
- *pulmonary angiography*
- *left ventricular ejection fraction measurement*

Cardiac disorders

Anthracyclines and anthracenediones

All the agents in this family—to a variable degree—have cumulative myocardial toxicity that may lead to cardiac insufficiency.

Cardiotoxicity is associated with some important characteristics.

- Risk is increased with underlying cardiomyopathy; an evaluation of cardiac function must be made before treatment is initiated.
- Maximum doses have been defined as the risk increases exponentially with cumulative doses (Table 10): higher doses should not be given. However, as there is considerable variation between patients, cardiac function should be re-evaluated during treatment.
- Cardiac damage may not become apparent until a long time after treatment and therefore great care must be used in young patients with curable cancer.
- Risk can be potentiated with mediastinal irradiation.

Table 10 "Maximum" cumulative doses of the most commonly used anthracyclines (beyond these doses cardiotoxicity is very likely to occur)

Doxorubicin	500 mg/m^2
Epirubicin	900 mg/m^2
Idarubicin	180 mg/m^2
Mitoxantrone	160 mg/m^2
Pirarubicin	700 mg/m^2

Measurement of ventricular ejection fraction by isotope scintigraphy is the most useful investigation:

- for diagnosis of pre-existing myocardial disease before initiating chemotherapy
- for follow-up of cardiac function when the dose is near to the maximum tolerated.

An alternative would be an echocardiographic study of left ventricular function.

Other agents

5-fluorouracil

Cardiotoxicity occurs when there is:

- pre-existing ischemic heart disease
- use of a continuous IV infusion; complications tend to occur during the first treatment cycles and may consist of angina and life-threatening arrhythmias.

The onset of chest pain in a patient receiving 5-fluorouracil calls for:

- immediate cessation of the infusion
- a GTN (glyceryl trinitrate) test
- emergency ECG and cardiac investigations.

Cyclophosphamide, ifosfamide

Cardiotoxicity can occur:

- with the administration of single high dose of cyclophosphamide ($>50\,mg/kg$), for example as conditioning for bone marrow transplantation
- clinically, as fatal or reversible acute heart failure.

Ischemic heart disease

Early coronary artery disease is a complication arising with increasing frequency, after treatment of Hodgkin's lymphoma, especially in cases of mediastinal irradiation and in smokers.

Genital function abnormalities

It is essential that abnormalities of the genital functions are considered:

- in the follow-up of neoplasms curable by chemotherapy in young patients, particularly:
  - leukemia and solid tumors in children
  - lymphoma and Hodgkin's disease
  - testicular cancer
  - nonmetastatic breast cancer
- as soon as the cancer is diagnosed:
  - to choose certain treatments
  - to inform the patient and/or the family (children)
  - to take precautions for the future.

In men

Impotence

There is rarely a direct link with chemotherapy. Other explanations are:

- lesions of the Leydig cells: decrease of testosterone secretion and an increase in serum LH level
- psychogenic origin.

Infertility

Much more frequent, it may be due to several mechanisms:

- the disease itself: a number of patients present with oligo-asthenospermia before the cancer is treated, particularly in advanced states with general symptoms, so affecting the quality of the initial sperm sample;
- the treatments:
  - surgery: orchidectomy, retroperitoneal lymphadenectomy;
  - testicular irradiation (acute lymphold leukemia) or inverted Y irradiation;
  - chemotherapy, especially with alkylating agents able to induce permanent azoospermia (the MOPP regimen in Hodgkin's disease);
- age of the patient.

This infertility justifies—in cancers which are considered curable:

- freezing of sperm in any patient at or past puberty:
  - before the beginning of any treatment;
  - keeping informed the center where freezing is performed of the evolution of the disease;
  - except, at present, in HIV-positive patients.

These patients should be followed up with spermograms and FSH measurements every 6 months or until normal.

Pregnancy in partner

Pregnancy in the partner of any fertile patient should be advised against during chemotherapy to avoid the mutagenic risks of these treatments.

Although this time interval is arbitrary, a waiting period of two years after the end of treatment is most often recommended for two reasons:

- to have a more exact idea of the prognosis of the neoplasia;
- to allow complete resolution of the chromosomic lesions and the elimination, by maturation, of the spermatogonia present during chemotherapy.

Before puberty

In boys before puberty, the risk is at least as great as after puberty, as the reserve of spermatogonic cells is a great deal less.

Hormone levels do not allow monitoring of testicular lesions. It is therefore imperative that the family be completely informed.

In women

Fertility

Infertility caused by chemotherapy results from:

- direct lesions of the ovocytes (irreversible)
- indirect lesions of the cells of the follicular stroma (variable reversibility, sometimes very delayed).

Chemotherapy has no contraceptive action and should always be associated with adequate contraception.

Chemotherapy may induce: **ovarian dysfunction**, characterized by:

- clinically, phases of amenorrhea (with, possibly, hot flushes) alternating with unusually heavy or prolonged periods
- varying levels of serum FSH and LH and urinary estradiol.

Pregnancy remains possible at this stage.

This syndrome may evolve, either as a return to normal which may take several years after the stopping of chemotherapy, or towards an **early menopause**, with:

- clinically, prolonged amenorrhea and hot flushes
- an increase in FSH (over 15 U IU/L), in LH (over 45 U IU/L) and a decrease in plasma and urine levels of estradiol.

The frequency and severity of ovarian dysfunction depends upon:

- the age of the patient: the nearer the patient is to the menopause, the higher the frequency
- the type of drug (alkylating agents in particular) and the total dose administered:
  - busulfan over 150 mg/m^2;
  - mechlorethamine over 72 mg/m^2;
  - chlorambucil over 750 mg/m^2;
  - cyclophosphamide over an approximate dose of 20–25 g/m^2 under the age of 29, 6.3–9 g/m^2 from age 30 to 39, 3–6.5/m^2 after 39 and above all, risk of menopause if the treatment is continued after the onset of amenorrhea;
  - etoposide (especially after prolonged oral treatment);
  - cisplatin.

Before puberty

Chemotherapy:

- causes histological lesions of the ovaries
- most often does not jeopardize normal puberty and later pregnancies
- but can increase the likelihood of early menopause.

Teratogenicity

In principle, there should be a waiting period of two years between the end of treatment by chemotherapy or irradiation, and conception.

With rare exceptions (vinblastine), the teratogenicity of cytotoxic drugs justifies:

- not prescribing them during the first trimester of pregnancy
- the proposal of a therapeutic termination of pregnancy in case of administration by mistake during the first trimester of pregnancy.

However, the risk of fetal malformation after maternal anticancer chemotherapy is only slightly increased. The value of systematic amniocentesis is under discussion.

Skin reactions

Alopecia

Alopecia appears 3–6 weeks after therapy is started.

Its severity depends upon the drugs used.

Severe alopecia
Doxorubicin
Epirubicin
Cyclophosphamide at high doses
Ifosfamide
Etoposide

Mild or no alopecia
5-fluorouracil
Vincristine
Vinblastine
Vindesine
Cisplatin
Carboplatin
Mitoxantrone
Methotrexate

Alopecia can be prevented or limited:

• by avoiding hair treatments during chemotherapy
• by cooling the scalp during the perfusion of antimitotics with a cap specifically designed for the purpose:
  – of varying efficacy; requires correct, professional installation
  – not to be used for certain diseases: hemopathies, cutaneous metastases.

Acroparesthesia

Certain anticancer drugs (bleomycin, vinca alkaloids), may be responsible for persistent, possibly permanent, acrosyndromes.

Allergic reactions

Certain anti-cancer drugs may cause various cutaneous reactions (urticaria, erythema multiforme), particularly:

• asparaginase
• bleomycin
• teniposide.

Cytosine arabinoside at high doses or in prolonged continuous intravenous administration may provoke palmar and plantar desquamation, in sheets.

14 Adverse drug reactions in HIV-seropositive patients

Christian Bénichou, Muriel Eliaszewicz and Antoine Flahault

Introduction

Patients infected with the human immunodeficiency virus (HIV) will receive, after a certain stage of the disease, a number of drugs. Some of them are intended to directly fight the HIV infection itself, others to avoid or treat its complications. In these patients, adverse drug reactions are unusual in their frequency, not in their type. They may involve all the systems, as does the viral infection itself or its complications. They reduce the already limited therapeutic possibilities. Thus they modify the usual management of certain drug reactions in immunocompetent patients.

The description and the study of adverse drug reactions in patients who are HIV seropositive are vital to facilitate their detection and their prevention. They may also provide better comprehension of the mechanisms responsible for adverse drug reactions occurring in immunocompetent patients. HIV infection is undoubtedly a model for a study of drug safety, as the frequency of reactions is particularly high and the clinical or biological background of occurrence particularly well documented. The incidence of certain reactions, such as skin reactions, generally considered as indicating hypersensitivity, makes them as frequent as the dose-dependent, pharmacological reactions. It is probably useful, from this perspective, to compare HIV-seropositive patients undergoing an adverse reaction with reaction-free patients at the same stage of infection, with patients at different stages of infection, with populations infected by other viruses (EBV, CMV) or with other immunodeficient states of drug or nondrug origin and, finally, with immunocompetent populations.

Drugs are able to induce clinical or biological abnormalities that cannot be differentiated from abnormalities of nondrug origin. Follow-up of HIV-infected patients has shown that the association of certain diseases with certain drugs increases the risk of drug reactions. The search for an enhancing, synergistic or at least a nonneutralizing mechanism may improve the knowledge or the prevention of all adverse drug reactions.

Adverse Drug Reactions. A Practical Guide to Diagnosis and Management. Edited by C. Bénichou.
©1994 John Wiley & Sons Ltd.

The spread of HIV infection, the attempt to maintain the infected patient at home in a normal life as long as possible and the frequency of adverse drug reactions mean that any physician is likely to be confronted with the diagnosis and treatment of a drug-related toxicity in an HIV-positive patient. It is useful therefore to make as complete a review as possible of the different toxicities observed with the drugs most often employed in this illness.

On 28 May 1993, a certain number of physicians specializing in the treatment of HIV infection and/or adverse drug reactions, met to discuss a document* which had been previously communicated to all the participants. This document was completed or modified during the meeting. Consensus was not the main objective, given the recent and changing nature of knowledge in this field. However, the description, the incidences and the recommendations which are presented here reflect the opinion of a large majority—and often the unanimity—of the participants concerning the cutaneous, hematologic, hepatic and gastrointestinal reactions discussed during this meeting. They will be followed by other reactions that were not discussed during the meeting.

---

*The preparation of this document and the organization of this meeting are the work of Dr Muriel Eliaszewicz, from the Institut Pasteur Hospital, Paris, in collaboration with the Pharmacovigilance Department of Roussel Uclaf, Paris.

The list of participants is as follows:
Christian Bénichou, M.D. (Pharmacovigilance, Roussel Uclaf—Paris), Eric Caumes, M.D. (Hôpital de la Pitié-Salpétrière—Paris), Gaby Danan, M.D. (Pharmacovigilance, Roussel Uclaf—Paris), Professor Jean-François Delfraissy (Hôpital Antoine Béclère—Clamart), Professor Jean Dormont (Hôpital Antoine Béclère—Clamart), Professor Bertrand Dupont (Hôpital de l'Institut Pasteur—Paris), Muriel Eliaszewicz, M.D. (Hôpital de l'Institut Pasteur—Paris), Pierre-Marie Girard, M.D. (Hôpital Rothschild—Paris), Bruno Hoen, M.D. (Hôpital de Brabois—Nancy), Professor Catherine Leport (Hôpital Bichat Claude Bernard—Paris), Eric Oksenhandler, M.D. (Hôpital Saint-Louis—Paris), Jacques Reynes, M.D. (Hôpital Gui de Chauliac—Montpellier), Professor Jean-Claude Roujeau (Hôpital Henri Mondor—Créteil), Philippe Saiag, M.D. (Hôpital Ambroise Paré—Boulogne), Philippe Solal-Céligny, M.D. (Clinique Victor Hugo—Le Mans).

Skin and/or mucosal reactions

A skin reaction

Description

In the majority of cases, it consists of an erythematous maculopapulous rash, spreading from head to foot, with rare pruritus. The rash disappears in 3–5 days, with no sequelae.

Less frequent reactions have been reported such as vasculitis, fixed drug eruption and increased skin pigmentation.

Signs of severity

Signs of severity are **initial urticarial eruption** or occurrence of **mucosal lesions** and/or **skin detachments**, such as those seen in Stevens–Johnson syndrome or TEN. A burning sensation and/or a fever over 40°C lasting more than 48 hours are also warning signs.

*The **incidence** of these **severe reactions** is likely to be **higher** than in the general population.*

Drugs involved

Antibacterial sulfonamides

A high incidence of rashes in HIV patients treated with high doses of cotrimoxazole has been reported during the treatment of *Pneumocystis carinii* pneumonia: 40–60% of HIV patients had a reaction, vs 0 out of 15 immunocompromised non-HIV-infected patients, and 3–4% of immunocompetent patients treated at usual dosage. These reactions seem to be less frequent when in case of severe decrease of CD4 and CD8.

At a dose of 800 mg/day, cotrimoxazole induces a cutaneous reaction in 10% of HIV-infected patients.

Other sulfonamides given in combination are also responsible for rashes:

- sulfadiazine + pyrimethamine (30–50%)
- sulfadoxine + pyrimethamine: a few cases have been reported.

It seems illogical to use this combination, with which some severe cases have been reported.

Other drugs

- Dapsone + trimethoprim: 13% of patients
- Dapsone + pyrimethamine for prevention: 9% of patients
  Pyrimethamine alone (50 mg/3 per week): 8–10%
- Clindamycin + pyrimethamine: 20–50% of patients
- Amoxicillin (mostly in association with clavulanic acid)

The increased incidence of cutaneous reactions seems to be related to the CD4 count: it reaches 63% when the CD4 count is below 200/μg/L, vs 10% when the CD4 count is over 200/μg/L, and 3–10% in immunocompetent patients.

- Anti-tuberculosis agents: 10% for the combination rifampicin, pyrazinamide, isoniazid, ethambutol and 20% for thiacetazone

Pyrazinamide is often combined with allopurinol, which can be responsible for drug eruptions.

- Bleomycin: 10–20% of patients

  And also phenobarbitone, phenytoin, carbamazepine, quinolones, foscarnet, ganciclovir, interferon, DDI (didanosine), clofazimine (cutaneous pigmentation) and atovaquone.

Skin reactions do not seem to be more frequent in patients given AZT (zidovudine) than in controls.

Evidence implicating a drug

Time to onset: the rash appears 8–12 days after the beginning of the treatment, and sooner if the patient has been previously sensitized. It can also appear later, particularly for prophylactic dosages.

The symptoms are not helpful for diagnosis, since pruritus, usual in drug-induced rashes, is a very common complaint in HIV patients.

It is because these reactions are common that the drugs are usually suspected.

Management

If there are no signs of severity, and no effective alternative drug, it is reasonable to continue the suspected drug(s), because these reactions may be short-lived, even if the drug is continued.

A reduction in dosage sometimes permits the critical period to be overcome.

Desensitization protocols are currently being evaluated.

In approximately 5–30% of cases, the drug has to be stopped since signs of severity appear.

As for cotrimoxazole, after nonserious reactions occurring at prophylactic dosages, reintroduction may be tried, mainly if there is no more efficient alternative drug.

It has not been proved that corticosteroids can influence the occurrence of a skin reaction. Indeed, comparing the groups with and without corticosteroids is generally biased as, in the available series, patients are under corticosteroid therapy for other indications than the prevention of a skin reaction.

Mucosal reactions

Three types of mucosal reactions have been described, with different localizations depending on the drug:

Ulcerations

In the mouth (aphtosis may be suspected): alpha interferon, DDC (zalcitabine). Mouth ulcerations related to interferon are the most serious and may lead to cessation of treatment.

Numerous other causes must be searched for: HSV or CMV infections, HIV-induced aphta, lymphomas, etc.

In the esophagus: AZT, foscarnet (15%).

Recommend taking AZT with a sufficient quantity of liquids and avoiding subsequent long periods of lying down.

On the external genitalia: foscarnet.

Antiseptic cleaning and drying of the genital mucosa after each micturition may permit a trial reintroduction.

Pigmentation in the mouth

This has been described with AZT, which may be continued with no consequences.

Early Kaposi's sarcoma may be suspected.

Candidiasis

Generally related to the disease, this may be induced by repeated courses of antibiotics or corticosteroids.

Management

Stopping the drugs inducing the candidiasis is often sufficient to improve the local infection.

However, a local or systemic antifungal treatment sometimes becomes necessary to cure the infection and may occasionally be given preventively.

Hair, nails, teeth

- Linear melanonychia: AZT
- Ciliary hypertricosis: AZT

This drug may be continued with no consequences.

Hematological reactions

Introduction

HIV-infected patients may already have abnormal hematological values before any treatment is instituted. This is because the HIV has a double adverse effect:

- on the bone marrow: stem cells, abnormal maturation, lack of growth factors
- peripheral: immune mechanisms.

The hematological disorders are rarely confined to one type of blood cell. For those patients receiving several concomitant drugs, logical management is to try to continue the most potent antiinfectious therapy.

Anemia

Definition

An asymptomatic HIV-infected patient is generally anemic. For a symptomatic patient, the Hb value before treatment is often close to 10 g/dL. In the absence of clinical signs of poor tolerance, fall of 25% of the initial value necessitates a change in management strategy.

For an immunocompetent patient, anemia is defined by an Hb value below 12 g/dL for a female and 13 g/dL for a male.

Signs of poor tolerance

Dyspnea, fatigue, vertigo, tinnitus, postural hypotension, headaches.

Evidence implicating a drug

The time to onset can vary according to the mechanism of the anemia, and is therefore not very indicative.

A drug-induced origin is more likely if the hematological anomaly:

- is **reversible** in a few weeks when the doses are reduced or the medication stopped;
- **occurs again** after the reintroduction of the drug, which may be tried after eliminating a hemolytic mechanism.

*In cases of bi- or pancytopenia, especially with fever, a **bone marrow biopsy** may reveal an infection with mycobacteria, leishmania, toxoplasma or a bone marrow disorder. The biopsy is not so useful for the diagnosis of microbiological infections. But it may show a megaloblastic marrow demonstrating a deficiency in folic acid.*

Features according to drug

Anemia is often related to AZT

For doses of 500–600 mg, the incidence would be about 30% for AIDS patients.

Anemia is:

- dose-dependent
- macrocytic or normocytic
- nonregenerative
- dependent on the stage of the disease and better tolerated at the beginning.

Macrocytosis helps confirm treatment compliance and does not itself require any treatment.

Anemia may occur at any time during treatment. It appears generally in the second month, when it often becomes severe enough to require stopping the drug.

Other drugs

- Dapsone: the anemia is hemolytic and dose-dependent. A deficit in G6PD is to be searched for in high-risk groups.
- Chemotherapy: rarely affects only the red cells.
- Rarely: foscarnet, GM-CSF.
- Pyrimethamine: isolated anemia, corrected by folinic acid.

A methemoglobinemia above 10% has been seen in 36% of patients: it is dose-dependent and requires stopping or reducing the drug if it is above 10%.

Management

Well-standardized for AZT

- Temporary suspension of the drug if Hb < 7.5 g/dL, or drops more than 2 g in 1 month. The reintroduction should be gradual.
- If the Hb is between 7.5 and 9 g/dL, the dose may be halved.

Blood transfusions may be necessary if the drug must be continued in the absence of alternative therapies.

This strategy is a general guide for the other types of anemia involving drugs.

Neutropenia

Definition

For asymptomatic HIV patients, neutropenia is frequent and the threshold to modify the treatment is 1000/μg/L.

Neutropenia, in the immunocompetent patient, is defined by a number of polymorphonuclear neutrophils (PN) less than 1500/μL (1.5 × 10⁹/L).

Signs of severity

Neutropenia is considered as severe when the PN count is less than 500/μL (0.5 × 10⁹/L).

The bacterial superinfections of severe neutropenia are more frequent with a lower count and have a longer duration. Except with a very low count, a reduction in the dosage is often sufficient to allow continuation of the drug.

Evidence implicating a drug

The occurrence of an acute and isolated neutropenia (without anemia or thrombocytopenia) will weigh in favor of a drug-related origin. Reversibility is less total and is slower than in the immunocompetent patient.

Specific pattern according to drug

The main groups of agents mostly involved are:

- **AZT:** neutropenia is dose-dependent, and usually starts after several months of treatment, with a progressive deterioration;
- **Folinic acid antagonists:**
  - trimethoprim, pyrimethamine: neutropenia is dose- and duration-dependent;
  - sulfonamides (cotrimoxazole, sulfadiazine, sulfadoxine);
- **ganciclovir:** 30% of patients;
- **antitumoral chemotherapies:** in order of increasing toxicity: bleomycin,

At a dose of 500–600 mg/day, the neutropenia appears in 37% of AIDS patients, as opposed to 2% of asymptomatic HIV-infected patients.

30–50% of AIDS patients and 8% of other immunodeficient patients are affected.

vincristine, velbe, VP 16 and adriamycin
- **antibiotics**, principally beta-lactamines.

Other drugs are less commonly involved:

- Interferons, clindamycin, foscarnet, pentamidine, rifampicin, DDI.

Rifampicin-induced neutropenias commonly have an immunologic mechanism.

Management

Well-standardized for AZT:

- Transient suspension of treatment when the PN count is below 750/µg/L (confirmed by two samples). The drug is reintroduced progressively with increasing dosage.

A reduction in the dosage and a close monitoring of the count may be enough if the count is between 750 and 1000/µg/L.

Other drugs

- Antitumoral chemotherapies may benefit from combination with growth factor (G-CSF or GM-CSF) to reduce the duration of neutropenia.

The expected benefit of these drugs in reducing the incidence of superinfections is yet to be proven.

- Systemic ganciclovir may be replaced by intravitreous injections for neutropenic patients, or by foscarnet.

This mode of administration is used exclusively for CMV retinitis. Growth factors are used by some with ganciclovir; the innocuity on viral replication is established for G-CSF but not for GM-CSF.

- Folinic acid may be added to prophylactic regimen using high doses of cotrimoxazole.

Most of the time these adjustments will not be enough to control the neutropenia and a reduction in doses or a definite cessation of the offending drug is necessary if the white cell count remains below 750/µg/L. The threshold is reduced to 500/µg/L if there is no therapeutic alternative.

Thrombocytopenia

Definition

Thrombocytopenia is defined by a platelet count $< 100\,000/\mu g/L$.

Specific drug-induced disorders

The two main types of drugs are

- **folic acid antagonists** (sulfonamides and pyrimethamine). Thrombocytopenia occurs in approximately 15% of patients, as opposed to 1% in immunocompetent patients.

- **ganciclovir:** in 5% of the patients.

Thrombocytopenia induced by GM-CSF, AZT and foscarnet is exceptional.

Management

- It is rare that even a very low platelet count induces bleeding, even in HIV-infected patients. The suspected drug(s) should be stopped if the platelet count is below $50\,000/\mu g/L$. In the case of hemorrhage, platelet transfusions are required.

If the platelet count remains above $50\,000/\mu g/L$, it is not always necessary to stop the drug in the absence of hemorrhage and when there is no therapeutic alternative. Close monitoring is necessary. Folinic acid may be added to prophylactic regimen using high doses of cotrimoxazole and in malnourished patients.

Table 1 Principal drugs inducing blood cytopenia

Anemia	Neutropenia	Thrombocytopenia	Eosinophilia
AZT	AZT	Folic acid antag.	GM-CSF
Cytotoxic drugs	Folic acid antag.	Ganciclovir	Sulfonamides
Dapsone (hemolysis)	Ganciclovir	Cytotoxic drugs	
Foscarnet	Interferon	GM-CSF	
GM-CSF (hemolysis)	Cytotoxic drugs	Rifampicin	
Amphotericin	Clindamycin		
5FC (5-fluorocytosine)	Rifampicin		
	DDI		
	5FC		
	Amphotericin		
	Beta-lactamines		

Liver test abnormalities

It is difficult to ascertain the role of a drug suspected in a liver test abnormality, because of the high incidence, in HIV-infected patients, of viral hepatitis or liver granulomatosis induced by infections or tumors. Overall, a drug-induced liver abnormality is found in 10–20% of patients.

The drugs mainly responsible are:

- Sulfonamides
- Isoniazid
- Ketoconazole
- Clarithromycin
- AZT
- Interferons
- Growth factors
- Valproic acid

Sulfonamide-induced hepatotoxicity often appears at the same time as a skin reaction, usually 8–12 days after the beginning of the treatment.

The arguments relating to the diagnosis of a drug-related origin have already been described in the relevant chapter.

Management

Hepatocellular damage (marked increase in aminotransferases)

The management depends on the baseline values of aminotransferases:

- If the liver function tests are normal before the treatment, the drug(s) should be stopped when the ALT value is above **3 times** the upper limit of the normal range.

  When several drugs may be suspected, the drug considered as the most hepatotoxic should be withdrawn first when the threshold is reached.

- If there are abnormal liver function tests before the beginning of therapy, the suspected drug(s) may be continued as long as ALT values are less than **5 times** the upper limit of the normal value. A higher value imposes stopping the drug(s).

  Chronic hepatitis (B and/or C) is the usual cause of abnormal baseline liver function tests.

Cholestatic damage (predominant increase of alkaline phosphatases)

An **increase in alkaline phosphatases**, irrespective of its value, does not require the discontinuation of the treatment if it is necessary for the patient, except:

*A baseline raised level of alkaline phosphatases is most often due to a **granulomatosis**, an **infection** or a **sclerosing cholangitis**.*

- in the case of jaundice;
- if the increase of aminotransferases, usually associated with cholestasis, reaches the above mentioned thresholds.

Gastrointestinal reactions

Nausea and vomiting

All the drugs received can cause nausea and vomiting in HIV-infected patients, mainly because the doses used are higher and drug combinations more frequent than in seronegative patients.

- Sulfonamides (cotrimoxazole and sulfadiazine mainly) can cause these reactions in up to 50% of patients, sometimes requiring stopping the drug.
- Macrolides and related drugs (clindamycin).
- Atovaquone

Management

- Try antiemetics, even in injectable form if necessary.
- Change the mode of oral administration (fragmented doses) or inject the drug if suitable.
- In some cases, stopping the drug and looking for alternatives is the only possibility.

If the vomiting persists, an organic intracerebral cause (such as intracranial hypertension) or a digestive tract disorder (such as esophageal candidiasis, extrinsic compression or stenosis of pylorus) should be excluded.

Diarrhea

Diarrhea exists in 50–90% of AIDS patients. A drug intolerance is therefore difficult to identify.

Management of diarrhea, occurring in a patient within 1 month after the beginning of the treatment, depends on whether the patient is febrile or not.

Diarrhea associated with fever

Endoscopic and microbiological investigations can identify some common pathogens.

The most frequently isolated organisms are salmonellas, atypical mycobacteria, CMV, etc.

Pseudomembranous colitis (PMC)
The presence of *Clostridium difficile* (CD) in the stools may be a sign of PMC if the patient has fever, but fever may not be present. Among drug-induced PMC, *antibiotics* are the main causative agents. Long and repeated treatments may increase the incidence. **Clindamycin** is the highest risk for these patients, who tend not to be prescribed broad-spectrum antibiotics.

A Clostridium difficile induced diarrhea is not synonymous with PMC in these patients needing long and repeated hospitalization, during which the microorganism is nosocomial and epidemic in nature.

Management

- Stop the suspected drug(s).
- Identify *Clostridium difficile* and/or its toxin.
- Ideally, perform sigmoidoscopy or colonoscopy if the status of the patient permits it.
- Give oral vancomycin or metronidazole.

Most isolated CD belong to the C subgroup and almost 100% of those are toxinogens.

Diarrhea without fever

- Look repeatedly for parasites in the stools.
- If no parasites are found, the diarrhea, of recent occurrence or aggravation, may be a simple **antibiotic-induced diarrhea**, which usually subsides when the antibiotic is stopped.

The most frequent are cryptosporides, microsporides, giardia, isospora belli.

Some excipients (e.g. in DDI) may induce diarrhea.

Abdominal pain

Steroids

High doses are given in these patients but steroids rarely cause gastrointestinal pain.

Pancreatitis

The incidence of drug-induced pancreatitis is unknown because of a lack of epidemiological studies on this reaction.

Nondrug causes are dominated by CMV, mycobacterias and toxoplasma.

The drugs mainly involved are:

- pentamidine
- DDI
- DDC

A few cases have also been reported with:

- sulfonamides
- steroids
- cyclines
- paracetamol
- opioids.

Management

Most of the drug-induced pancreatitis in HIV-infected patients are asymptomatic, and found during systemic biological monitoring.

The drug(s) should be suspended if typical abdominal pain is associated with an increase in blood amylase and/or lipase.

Mechanisms of toxicity include:

- *direct cellular toxicity*
- *arteriolar thrombosis*
- *spasm of the canal of Wirsung.*

In the absence of clinical symptoms, increase in blood amylase in a patient treated with IV pentamidin or DDI, the monitoring, particularly for lipase, must be intensified.

Renal failure

There are two types of renal disorders in HIV-infected patients, secondary to different mechanisms (dehydration, sepsis, opportunistic infections and the HIV itself):

- **Acute** renal failure: secondary to hypovolemia, or intrinsic due to acute tubular necrosis, interstitial nephritis or tubular obstruction by crystals;
- **Chronic progressive** renal failure, mainly due to a glomerular disease, possibly caused by the virus itself.

Drug-induced nephrotoxicity

Known nephrotoxic drugs	Potentially nephrotoxic drugs
Amphotericin B	Cotrimoxazole
IV Pentamidine	Rifampicin
Foscarnet	Acyclovir
Sulfadiazine	Dapsone
Aminoglycosides	
X-ray contrast media	

Usual mechanisms:

- *Amphotericin B: tubular disease, reduction in glomerular filtration rate, cylinder formation;*
- *Pentamidine: tubular insufficiency due to the renal accumulation of pentamidine;*
- *Foscarnet: tubular necrosis;*
- *Sulfadiazine: crystals in urine in the case of acidic pH.*

Management

- A drug-induced mechanism should always be suspected in a case of **acute** renal failure.
- Depending on the drug, some specific preventive measures should be taken: IV saline hydration (1.5 L/24 h) for foscarnet; alkalinization of urine (pH should be >7.5).
- In the case of renal failure, the suspected drug(s) should be stopped.

For the other drugs, adequate hydration is also mandatory for these hypovolemic patients.

In the case of renal failure, there are other toxic manifestations associated

If the infection is severe, and there are no alternative drugs, the drug(s) may be continued with reduced dosage (every other day infusion of pentamidine and amphotericin B) with close laboratory monitoring of diuresis and renal function. The doses of the other drugs should be reduced accordingly, if they are eliminated via the kidney.

with acute pentamidine toxicity (pancreatitis, hypoglycemia, etc.). Liposomal presentation for amphotericin B may improve tolerance to the drug.

Metabolic disorders

Metabolic disorders are often symptomatic, sometimes life threatening, and may need urgent correction.

Hypocalcemia

Foscarnet-induced hypocalcemia has been described (formation of ionized foscarnet-calcium complex). Ketoconazole can also be involved (interference with the synthesis of 1,25 dihydroxyvitamin D). The incidence of hypocalcemia with foscarnet is influenced by the speed of infusion, which should take longer than 90 minutes. Good hydration and calcium supplements are essential preventive measures. Foscarnet should only be started after checking the patient's renal function and metabolic status.

Hypokalemia/hypomagnesemia

They have been described with foscarnet (tubular disease) and amphotericin B.

Hypoglycemia, sometimes followed by hyperglycemia

They have been described with IV pentamidine (beta pancreatic cell toxicity), cotrimoxazole or DDI. Of patients treated with pentamidine, 57% have abnormal glycemia.

IV pentamidine-induced hypoglycemia occurs most often in patients treated with high doses, and with a degree of renal failure. The hypoglycemia must be corrected urgently, and pentamidine (with a long half-life) stopped immediately. However, if the *Pneumocystis* infection is severe, and there are no satisfactory alternatives, the treatment may be completed by reducing the dose (infusion every other day), and continuous round-the-clock checking of glucose levels.

Hyperuricemia

This has been described with pyrazinamide.

Endocrine disorders

Adrenal failure has been described in association with:

- rifampicin, phenytoin, opioids, with increased cortisol catabolism;
- ketoconazole, by inhibition of gluco- and androgenic steroids, with reduction of libido and gynecomastia;
- discontinuation of systemic steroid therapy: a progressive reduction of the dose is recommended after prolonged therapy, e.g. for thrombocytopenia.

Cardiac disorders

Cyclophosphamide and doxorubicin may induce a myocardial disorder, and require monitoring with a 3-monthly echocardiogram during long-term therapy.

Pentamidine may induce ventricular arrhythmias, torsades de pointe or cardiovascular collapse. This justifies continuous monitoring with ECG and blood pressure.

Amphotericin B may induce ventricular arrhythmias.

The metabolic disorders described above may also induce cardiac dysrhythmias.

Neurologic manifestations

CNS disorders (convulsions, confusional states)

They have been described with DDI, DDC, foscarnet, isoniazid and AZT.

In case of repeated convulsions (at least two separate episodes), and after elimination of an organic intracerebral lesion, anticonvulsants are justified with continuation of the offending drug if judged necessary. If the convulsions continue despite the anticonvulsants, the drug should be stopped and the blood levels of anticonvulsants checked. Phenobarbitone is to be avoided because of its powerful enzyme induction potential.

Peripheral and/or muscular disorders

Polyneuritis, mainly sensory, has been described with isoniazid, DDI and DDC. Neurogenic muscular disorders are seen with AZT. As muscular disorders have been described in the absence of AZT, and as some patients are able to take the drug again without reactions, the reintroduction of the drug can be tried, but it should be stopped again if the same reaction occurs at doses below 300 mg.

High-dose vitamins and adjustments of the drug dosage usually control a peripheral neuropathy. The drug may need to be stopped because of the clinical consequences: a progressive reintroduction may be allowed if there are no alternative drugs. The differential diagnosis between a neurologic or a muscular disorder is based on clinical course, muscular enzyme levels (CPK-aldolase), electromyography and, when necessary, muscle biopsy.

Hyperpyrexia

Isolated febrile reactions may be seen in the first days of treatment with IV amphotericin B, bleomycin, interferons, growth factors and pyrazinamide.

The pathophysiological mechanism for amphotericin B and bleomycin may be via the activation of pyrogenic cytokines.

Stopping the treatment for 2–3 days brings the temperature down and constitutes a diagnostic test, particularly if, on restarting the drug the fever starts again.

Effects on the immune system

Steroids, cytotoxic drugs and opioids have a deleterious effect on the immune system.

Opioids have three different actions on the immune system:

- Binding to membrane **peripheral receptors**, and therefore impairing phagocytic functions and cell immunity;
- Activation of **central opioid receptors** with stimulation of endogenous steroids;
- Action on the **sympathetic nervous system** with increased noradrenaline production, in itself an immunosuppressant.

IV drug abusers are particularly susceptible to infections (bacterial and fungal).

Prophylactic treatment of opportunistic infections (*Pneumocystis*) is justified in association with cytotoxic and steroid treatment.

Vaccination for HIV-infected patients

There are two potential problems:

- Would vaccinations cause a nonspecific and deleterious stimulation of the immune system? The current answer is no, and the usual timing of vaccinations is respected in HIV-infected patients (see box below).
- Would these immunosuppressed patients tolerate vaccination less well? All **inactivated** vaccines can be administered to HIV-infected patients, with the usual precautions.

For **live** vaccines, the contraindications are relative and should be tailored individually:

- **BCG:** The risk is inducing active, possibly lethal, BCGitis. The vaccine is not used in developed countries; however, a child with a strong family history may be vaccinated. In Africa, with the endemic local status, vaccination is recommended, regardless of the mother's HIV status.
- **Measles–Mumps–Rubella** is given to HIV-infected children, unless the AIDS syndrome is already severe (febrile hepatosplenomegaly), which is the case in less than 10% of neonatal patients.
- **Yellow fever** vaccination is justified if the patient **must** go to an endemic region. The vaccine is well tolerated, as long as the CD4 count is >200.
- **Live oral polio** vaccine has almost been discontinued in France and replaced by the injectable inactivated vaccine.

Inactivated vaccines with no risk	Live vaccines with restrictions
Injectable polio Diphtheria Tetanus Pneumococcal Rabies Meningococcal *Haemophilus influenzae* type b Injectable typhoid Hepatitis B Hepatitis A Flu Whooping cough	BCG Measles–Mumps–Rubella Yellow fever

The proposed calendar of vaccinations for an HIV-infected child is:

- Hepatitis B: birth–1 month–2 months
- Diphtheria–Tetanus–Whooping cough–Poliomyelitis and *Haemophilus*: 3–4–5 months
- Measles–Mumps–Rubella: 12 months
- Pneumococcal: 24 months.

References

Carr A, Swanson C, Penny R, et al. Clinical and laboratory markers of hypersensitivity to Trimethoprim-Sulfamethoxazole in patients with pneumocystis carinii pneumonia and AIDS. J Inf Dis 1993; 167: 180–5.

Cohen PT, Merle AS, Volberding PA. AIDS knowledge base. Waltham, Massachusetts, 1990.

Fischl MA, Parker CB, Pettinelli C, et al. A randomized controlled trial of a reduced daily dose of zidovudine in patients with the acquired immunodeficiency syndrome. N Engl J Med 1990; 323: 1009–14.

15 Management of adverse events during clinical trials

Christian Bénichou

Good Clinical Practices require the investigator to report to the sponsor serious adverse events occurring during clinical trials with a new drug but do not usually concern the management of these events. At the beginning of a clinical trial, little is known of the clinical tolerance of a new product, and when an abnormality appears the investigator must routinely envisage the possibility that it is caused by the drug. The first volunteers and patients to whom the product is administered are therefore closely monitored. They have agreed to participate in a trial, but the benefit they hope to gain, in comparison with available treatments, has obviously not yet been demonstrated. Therefore, for the different parties engaged in a clinical trial, it is essential to have the means of rapid detection of an abnormality and an assessment of the product's role. This explains the repetition of clinical and laboratory examinations in the trial protocols: the examinations must be frequent and the results of the laboratory workups analyzed from day to day. When hospitalized patients are involved, intensified monitoring is feasible, giving the investigator 24–48 hours to gather arguments for or against the continuation of treatment.

The principal questions that must be answered when an adverse event occurs are the following:

- **Is the abnormality caused by the product?** A drug-related origin must be accepted if sufficient evidence cannot be found for another satisfactory explanation, either a complication of the treated disease or another concomitant disease.
- **Is the likelihood of the abnormality enhanced by the personal characteristics of the patient?** The patient may have metabolic or kinetic characteristics that would explain or induce this abnormality, although the product could be well tolerated by other patients.
- **Should administration of the product to the patient be interrupted?** In principle this should be considered every time that the drug's role in the appearance of a potentially serious abnormality cannot be eliminated.

In addition, confronted with any new safety data, the sponsor must decide if it is legitimate to continue the development of the product. The answer will depend upon the nature and the incidence of the adverse events. Except in exceptional therapeutic classes, the incidence

---

Adverse Drug Reactions. A Practical Guide to Diagnosis and Management. Edited by C. Bénichou.
©1994 John Wiley & Sons Ltd.

acceptable for a severe reaction is very low. As the number of patients engaged in a clinical trial is limited, the first case or cases carry a considerable weight, and an error of interpretation may have serious consequences.

The investigator is responsible for the patient's wellbeing and must react quickly and correctly: he should immediately request a workup enabling him to answer the various questions raised. He must also rapidly take the decision to stop or continue the administration of the drug to the patient. Usually the investigator is a specialist in the treated condition, but he may not be familiar with all possible events outside his own domain. Thus he may not be aware of the potential risks in continuing administration of the study drug. Similarly, he may not be aware of the simple tests to be performed immediately in order to assess the role of the drug later on: it is necessary to seek the frequent causes of the abnormalities observed, and the individual metabolic and pharmacokinetic risk factors.

As reflection is preferable to improvisation, it seemed useful to prepare, with the help of specialists on adverse drug reactions in different fields, a series of flow charts illustrating the conduct recommended in the case of the occurrence of an abnormality during a clinical trial. Information collected at the time may allow specialists to assess later on the role of the product, using all available information.

Since 1987 we have been using a brochure containing recommendations, entitled "Guidelines for the management of clinical or laboratory abnormalities occurring during clinical trials." This brochure is explained and then presented to each investigator whenever a clinical trial is organized.

Description of the brochure

Seven potentially severe adverse events have been selected; most of them are laboratory abnormalities, but may later on be complicated by clinical manifestations. These are: neutropenia, thrombocytopenia, anemia, eosinophilia, increase in aminotransferases, acute renal failure, proteinuria and skin disorders.

For each abnormality, a precise definition is provided, generally drawn from the conclusions of national and international consensus meetings we have organized.

These definitions are based on elements that take into account the technical facilities available in hospital laboratories.

The procedure is presented in the form of a flow chart, which proposes either the continuation of therapy with intensive monitoring of which modalities are given in detail, or discontinuation of the study drug, which implies a list of investigations and a detailed follow-up. In addition, a special report form for each event must be filled out even if the role of the drug in initiating the event cannot be ascertained. This form is useful for the collection of the data resulting from patient questionnaires and diagnostic investigations carried out to detect non drug-related causes.

The attitudes recommended reflect the advice of experts, but they cannot be imposed. They cannot take the place of the investigator's own responsibility, particularly when it is a question of interrupting administration of the study drug. Nor can these recommendations be used as arguments for authority or responsibility *vis-à-vis* an administration or other industrial sponsors.

The recommendations apply only to the appearance of an abnormality which the patient did not present at entry into the trial. When pathological states already existing are aggravated, as in the case of a study of the tolerance of groups at risk, the investigator is more likely to be a specialist in the field concerned and is then completely competent to take the necessary decisions concerning the conduct of the treatment and the trial.

Comments

After several years of using this brochure, its objectives appear to have been fulfilled, at least partially. It is difficult to determine if the decrease in the number of cases assessed as "insufficiently documented" gives the true impact of these guidelines alone. Indeed, one should take into account the general improvement in the quality of clinical trials conducted during the last few years, and the increasing importance of the monitoring of drug safety. However, these procedures enable the sponsor to provide a better documented response to requests by health authorities concerning assessment of the study drug.

Certain guidelines and thresholds may appear to be arbitrary; they are, at least in part, based on the wide experience of experts in each medical field and specialists in charge of drug safety, who have participated in national or international consensus meetings on adverse drug reactions.

These guidelines constitute a valuable aid for all participants in clinical trials, to ensure suitable management in the case of adverse reactions. Each investigator pledges to do all that he can to perform all of the relevant tests and to fill out the specific forms. It is understood that these guidelines have been and will continue to be updated according to experience gained by use and the progress made in each medical field.

NEUTROPENIA

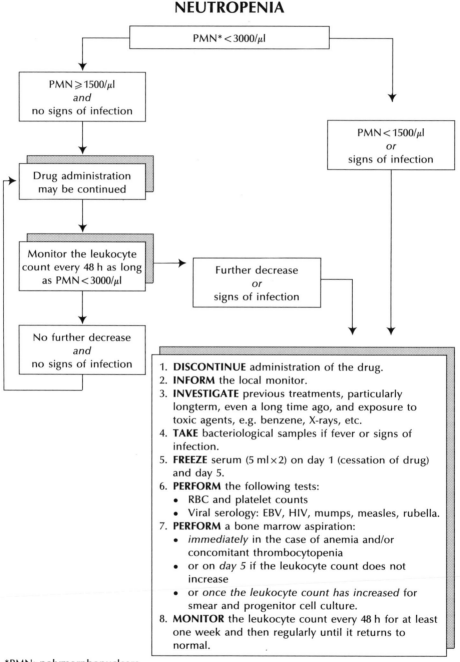

PMN* < 3000/μl

PMN ⩾ 1500/μl
and
no signs of infection

PMN < 1500/μl
or
signs of infection

Drug administration
may be continued

Monitor the leukocyte
count every 48 h as long
as PMN < 3000/μl

Further decrease
or
signs of infection

No further decrease
and
no signs of infection

1. **DISCONTINUE** administration of the drug.
2. **INFORM** the local monitor.
3. **INVESTIGATE** previous treatments, particularly longterm, even a long time ago, and exposure to toxic agents, e.g. benzene, X-rays, etc.
4. **TAKE** bacteriological samples if fever or signs of infection.
5. **FREEZE** serum (5 ml × 2) on day 1 (cessation of drug) and day 5.
6. **PERFORM** the following tests:
   • RBC and platelet counts
   • Viral serology: EBV, HIV, mumps, measles, rubella.
7. **PERFORM** a bone marrow aspiration:
   • *immediately* in the case of anemia and/or concomitant thrombocytopenia
   • or on *day 5* if the leukocyte count does not increase
   • or *once the leukocyte count has increased* for smear and progenitor cell culture.
8. **MONITOR** the leukocyte count every 48 h for at least one week and then regularly until it returns to normal.

*PMN: polymorphonuclears.
Reproduced with the permission of Roussel Uclaf.

EOSINOPHILIA

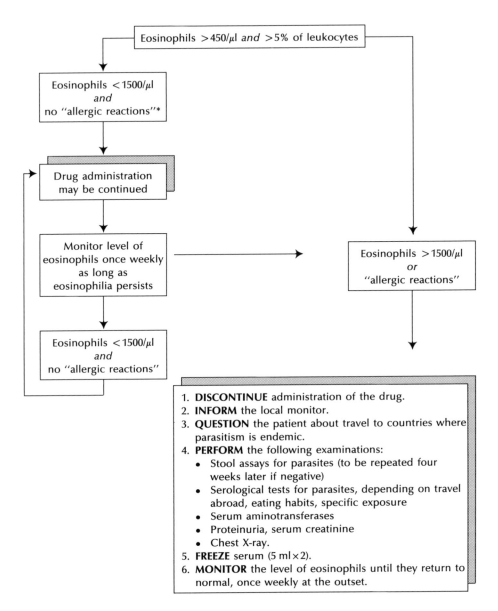

*"Allergic reactions" include: urticaria, angioedema, proteinuria, hepatitis, bronchospasm and fever.
Reproduced with the permission of Roussel Uclaf.

INCREASE IN AMINOTRANSFERASES*

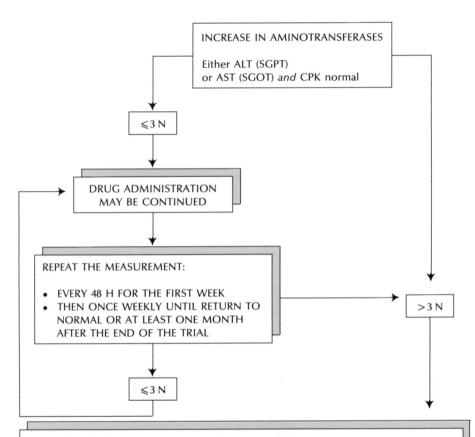

1. **DISCONTINUE** administration of the drug and **CHECK** the result immediately.
2. **INFORM** the local monitor.
3. **INTERVIEW** patient again about consumption of alcohol, drugs received *before* and *during* the trial and possible contamination by non-A, non-B virus in the last six months (blood or blood product transfusion, travel to Africa, Asia, intravenous drug addiction).
4. **INVESTIGATE FOR** illness and/or hypotension and/or episode of arrhythmia in the previous 48 h.

5. **FREEZE** serum (5 ml × 2).
6. **PERFORM** the following examinations:
   - Complete blood count
   - Serum creatinine
   - Anti-HAV IgM, anti-HB$_C$IgM, anti-HCV, anti-CMV IgM.
   Specific serologic markers of recent infection with:
   - EBV, Herpes viruses and toxoplasma (depending on the clinical context)
   - Hepatobiliary ultrasonography.
7. **MONITOR** aminotransferases every 48 h for the first week then once weekly until return to normal or for at least 3 months.

*Expressed as a multiple of the upper limit of normal (N) for the laboratory performing the assay.
Reproduced with the permission of Roussel Uclaf.

THROMBOCYTOPENIA

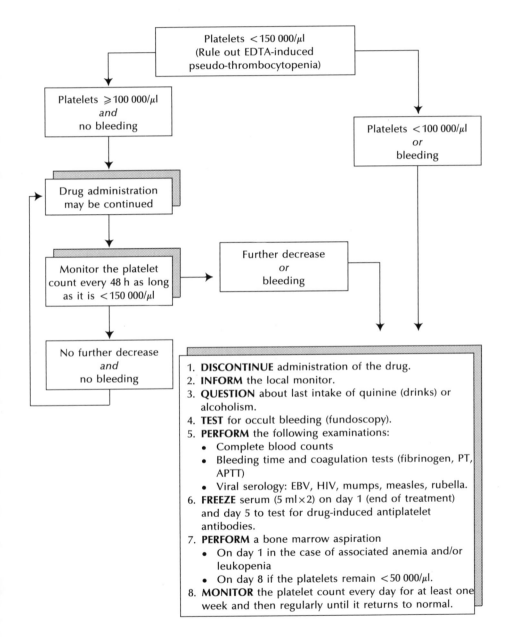

Platelets <150 000/μl
(Rule out EDTA-induced
pseudo-thrombocytopenia)

Platelets ≥100 000/μl
and
no bleeding

Platelets <100 000/μl
or
bleeding

Drug administration
may be continued

Monitor the platelet
count every 48 h as long
as it is <150 000/μl

Further decrease
or
bleeding

No further decrease
and
no bleeding

1. **DISCONTINUE** administration of the drug.
2. **INFORM** the local monitor.
3. **QUESTION** about last intake of quinine (drinks) or alcoholism.
4. **TEST** for occult bleeding (fundoscopy).
5. **PERFORM** the following examinations:
   • Complete blood counts
   • Bleeding time and coagulation tests (fibrinogen, PT, APTT)
   • Viral serology: EBV, HIV, mumps, measles, rubella.
6. **FREEZE** serum (5 ml×2) on day 1 (end of treatment) and day 5 to test for drug-induced antiplatelet antibodies.
7. **PERFORM** a bone marrow aspiration
   • On day 1 in the case of associated anemia and/or leukopenia
   • On day 8 if the platelets remain <50 000/μl.
8. **MONITOR** the platelet count every day for at least one week and then regularly until it returns to normal.

Reproduced with the permission of Roussel Uclaf.

ANEMIA

(Men: Hb<13 g/dl—Women: Hb<12 g/dl). Discontinue drug administration in all cases of acute and severe anemia

	MCV ≤ 80 fl	80 fl < MCV ≤ 105 fl	MCV > 105 fl
EXAMINATIONS	• SERUM IRON • TRANSFERRIN BINDING CAPACITY • FIBRINOGEN • HEMOGLOBIN ELECTROPHORESIS	RETICULOCYTE COUNT → INCREASED / DECREASED BILIRUBIN HAPTOGLOBIN BONE MARROW ASPIRATION BILIRUBIN INCREASED HAPTOGLOBIN DECREASED — NORMAL COOMBS' TEST (POSITIVE / NEGATIVE) TEST FOR ANTI-RBC AUTO-ANTIBODIES (indirect Coombs, Elution, Cold agglutinins) (POSITIVE / NEGATIVE) ANTI-DRUG ANTIBODIES (PRESENT / ABSENT) TEST FOR RBC ABNORMALITIES (POSITIVE)	• SERUM FOLATES • SERUM B12 • BONE MARROW ASPIRATION
DIAGNOSES	• IRON DEFICIENCY (Chronic bleeding) • INFLAMMATION • THALASSEMIA	• BONE MARROW HYPOPLASIA • AUTO-IMMUNE HEMOLYTIC ANEMIA (exceptionally drug-induced) • DRUG-INDUCED HEMOLYTIC ANEMIA • G6PD DEFICIENCY • SICKLE CELL ANEMIA • ACUTE HEMORRHAGE	• B12 DEFICIENCY • FOLATE DEFICIENCY • MALIGNANT HEMO—PATHIES

Reproduced with the permission of Roussel Uclaf.

PROTEINURIA

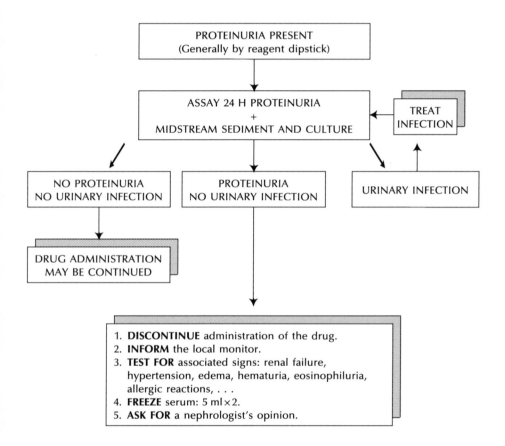

ACUTE RENAL FAILURE

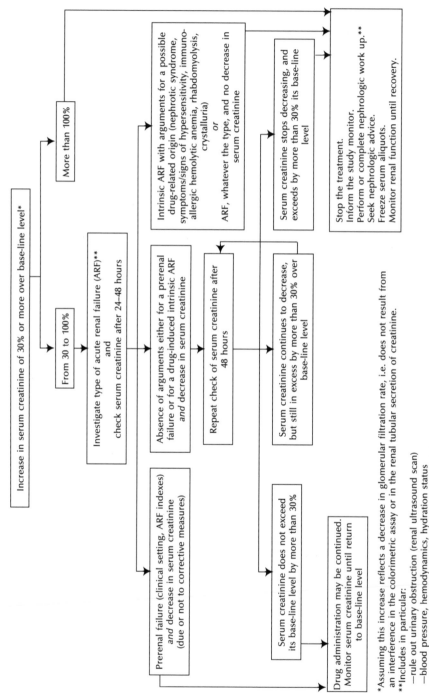

Increase in serum creatinine of 30% or more over base-line level*

From 30 to 100%

More than 100%

Prenatal failure (clinical setting, ARF indexes) *and* decrease in serum creatinine (due or not to corrective measures)

Investigate type of acute renal failure (ARF)** *and* check serum creatinine after 24-48 hours

Absence of arguments either for a prerenal failure or for a drug-induced intrinsic ARF *and* decrease in serum creatinine

Intrinsic ARF with arguments for a possible drug-related origin (nephrotic syndrome, symptoms/signs of hypersensitivity, immuno-allergic hemolytic anemia, rhabdomyolysis, crystalluria)

or

ARF, whatever the type, and no decrease in serum creatinine

Serum creatinine does not exceed its base-line level by more than 30%

Repeat check of serum creatinine after 48 hours

Serum creatinine continues to decrease, but still in excess by more than 30% over base-line level

Serum creatinine stops decreasing, and exceeds by more than 30% its base-line level

Drug administration may be continued. Monitor serum creatinine until return to base-line level

Stop the treatment.
Inform the study monitor.
Perform or complete nephrologic work up.**
Seek nephrologic advice.
Freeze serum aliquots.
Monitor renal function until recovery.

*Assuming this increase reflects a decrease in glomerular filtration rate, i.e. does not result from an interference in the colorimetric assay or in the renal tubular secretion of creatinine.
**Includes in particular:
—rule out urinary obstruction (renal ultrasound scan)
—blood pressure, hemodynamics, hydration status
—urinalysis (proteinuria, sediment with eosinophiluria), proteinemia
—indexes of ARF (see chapter 5)
—search for skin reaction
—liver tests, blood count with differential, creatine-kinase, crystalluria.

Reproduced with the permission of Roussel Uclaf.

PART II

Regulatory and Technical Issues

16 International reporting requirements for adverse drug events

Ernst Weidmann

The history of drug therapy is marked not only by therapeutic successes but also by failures due to the adverse effects of drugs. At an early stage this led to the question as to how drug safety can be assessed.

Paul Ehrlich, during the clinical development of salvarsan, asked for reports on adverse effects from all the doctors included in the clinical development and only after a thorough analysis allowed the distribution of the drug.

In the early 1960s, systems evolved that collected spontaneous reports on adverse reactions from doctors (see Mann RD, Pharmacoepidemiology and Drug Safety, 1992; 2: 215–24). Throughout the last 30 years these systems have demonstrated their usefulness in identifying and signaling rare and serious adverse events.

Based on this experience more and more regulatory authorities have asked for reporting of adverse reactions from national and international sources using the drug safety departments of the pharmaceutical companies as distributors. At the same time the WHO developed the WHO database, which is composed of reports from the respective country authorities. There was, and still is, a great difference in reporting requirements for adverse drug experiences or adverse reactions among the various countries.

Under the auspices of CIOMS, a working group of regulators and company experts has established definitions and procedures for handling adverse event reports from foreign countries. The results from this working group have been summarized in a format for suspected adverse reaction reports which hopefully will be adopted increasingly by health authorities world-wide.

Since expedited reporting might overload the health authorities of smaller countries and developing countries another CIOMS working party has developed a so-called safety update which can be consulted to gain a quick overview of the safety status of drugs using the single case documentation available within the pharmaceutical companies.

Adverse Drug Reactions. A Practical Guide to Diagnosis and Management. Edited by C. Bénichou.
©1994 John Wiley & Sons Ltd.

We have tried to summarize the worldwide reporting requirements by using the international network of local safety officers (LSOs) of the pharmaceutical division of Hoechst AG. The local safety officer is a person responsible in a specific country for all matters of drug safety. The corporate drug safety unit has been asked to supply their legal requirements and interpret them in accordance with the regulatory agencies in their countries. The result of these requests are presented in the following tables, which present the so-called strict requirements. This means that these countries require definite classes of adverse events in a given time frame; these contrast with worldwide requirements, which are sometimes less stringent and less well defined.

During the last decade reporting requirements have also been developed for products in clinical trials and under postmarketing surveillance. These are displayed in Tables 1–6.

Table 1 Strict* requirements for foreign case reports on marketed drugs from pharmaceutical companies[†]—All countries

Country	Time frame	Category
Australia	without delay	s/u
Austria	without delay	s/u
Canada	as soon as possible and within 15 working days of receipt	ns/u s/u
Denmark	immediately	s/u ns/u
Germany	without delay	ns/u
	without delay	s/u
Great Britain	immediately	s/u
Greece	within one month	all
Ireland	within 1–15 days	s/u
Italy	within 15 days of onset or 2 days from knowledge in company	s/u
Morocco	immediately	ns/u,l s/u, l
Netherlands	within 15 days	s/u s/l
Norway	immediately	s/u
Pakistan	15 days on receipt of report	ns/u, l s/u,l
Spain	within 15 days	ns/u, all s
Switzerland	new regulation under discussion	
Tanzania	immediately	ns/u s/u,l
USA	15 working days	s/u
Venezuela	immediately	ns/u, l s/u l

ns = non serious, s = serious, u = unlabeled, l = labeled
*0–30 days
[†]according to information given by LSOs

Table 2 Requirements for foreign case reports on marketed drugs*—All countries

Country	Time frame	Category
Argentina	none	none
Bangladesh	none	none
Belgium	none	none
Brazil	none	none
Chile	?	?
Columbia	none	none
Egypt	requirements under discussion	
Equador	in principle there are regulations, but ignored by companies and legal departments	
Finland	in principle, responsibility is on physicians and dentists	changes in the basic information
France	periodic safety reports 6-monthly during the 1st year, then yearly	all
Ghana	none	none
Guatemala	none	none
Hong Kong	none	none
India	none	none
Indonesia	none	none
Israel	none	none
Japan	none	none
Korea	no time frame	ns/u, l s/u, l
Malaysia	none	none
Mexico	none	none
Nigeria	without time frame	s/u, l
Peru	?	?
Philippines	none	none
Portugal	under discussion	?
Singapore	?	?
South Africa	only if an increased incidence or if an unexpected trend becomes apparent	s/u, l
Sri Lanka	none	none
Sweden	?	ns/u, all s (Guidelines)
Taiwan	none	none
Thailand	none	none
Turkey	none	none
Uruguay	none	none
Zaire	?	?
Zimbabwe	none	none

ns = non serious, s = serious, u = unlabelled, l = labelled
*according to information given by LSOs

Table 3 Strict* requirements for foreign adverse event reports from clinical trials†—All countries

Country	Time frame	Category	Causality
Austria	without delay	s/u	associated‡
Australia	without delay	s/u	associated
Canada	immediately	ns/u	
	immediately	s/u, e	
Denmark	as soon as possible after knowledge	s/u, e	associated
Finland	within 3–10 working days	s/u	associated
France	immediately	s/u, e	associated
Germany	without delay (after submission)	ns/u	associated
	without delay	s/u, e	associated
Great Britain	immediately	s/u, e	associated
Ireland	within 1–15 days	s/u, e	associated
Italy	within 15 days of onset or 2 days from knowledge	s/u	associated
Netherlands	within 15 days	s/u	
	within 30 days	s/e	
		ns/u, e	
Norway	immediately (within 15 days)	s/u, e	associated
Pakistan	15 days on receipt of report	ns/u, e	
		s/u, e	
Spain	within 15 days	ns/u	associated
		s/u, e	associated
	within 3 days	fatal/life-threatening	associated
Switzerland	without delay	s/u	associated
Tanzania	immediately	ns/u, e	
	immediately	s/u, e	
USA	10 days IND safety report ⎫ 15 days alert to NDA ⎭	s/u	associated

ns = non serious, s = serious, u = unexpected, e = expected
*0–30 days
†according to information given by LSOs
‡associated: a reasonable possibility of a causal relationship

Table 4 Requirements for foreign adverse event reports from clinical trials*—
All countries

Country	Time frame	Category	Causality
Argentina	none	none	
Bangladesh	none	none	
Belgium	none	none	
Brazil	none	none	
Chile	?	?	
Columbia	none	none	
Egypt	regulations in discussion		
Equador	no clear regulations		
Ghana	none	none	
Greece	none	none	
Guatemala	none	none	
Hong Kong	none	none	
India	?	s/u, e	
Indonesia	none	none	
Israel	none	none	
Japan		ns/u, e	associated[†]
		s/u, e	associated
Korea	no time frame	ns/u, e	associated
		s/u, e	associated
Malaysia	none	none	
Mexico	none	none	
Morocco	none	none	
Nigeria	without time frame	s/u, e	
Peru	?	?	
Philippines	none	none	
Portugal	under discussion	?	
Singapore	?	?	
South Africa	only if unexpected high incidence or a particular trend becomes apparent	s/u, e	
Sri Lanka	none	none	
Sweden	?	?	
Taiwan	none	none	
Thailand	none	none	
Turkey	none	none	
Uruguay	none	none	
Venezuela	upon receipt	ns/u, e	associated
	upon receipt	s/u, e	associated
Zaire	?	?	
Zimbabwe	none	none	

ns = non serious, s = serious, u = unexpected, e = expected
*according to information given by LSOs
[†]associated: a reasonable possibility of a causal relationship

Table 5 Strict* requirements for foreign adverse event reports from clinical observational monitoring projects (COMP)†—All countries

Country	Time frame	Category	Causality
Austria	without delay	s/u	associated‡
Australia	without delay	s/u	
Canada	as soon as possible and within	ns/u	
	15 working days of receipt	s/u	
Denmark	immediately	s/u	associated
Finland	within 3–10 working days	s/u, e	associated
France	immediately	s/u, e	associated
Germany	without delay	ns/u (1–49)	associated
	without delay	s/u, e	associated
Great Britain	immediately	s/u	associated
Ireland	within 1–15 days	s/u, e	associated
Morocco	immediately	ns/u, e	
	immediately	s/u, e	
Netherlands	within 15 days	s/u	
		s/e	
		ns/u, e	
Norway	immediately (within 15 days)	s/u, e	associated
Pakistan	15 days on receipt	ns/u, e	
		s/u, e	
Spain	within 15 days	ns/u	associated
		s/u, e	associated
	within 3 days	fatal/life-threatening	associated
Switzerland	new regulation under discussion	s/u	associated
Tanzania	immediately	ns/u, e	
	immediately	s/u, e	
USA	15 days alert to NDA	s/u	associated
Venezuela	upon receipt	ns/u, e	associated
	upon receipt	s/u, e	

ns = non serious, s = serious, u = unexpected (unlabeled), e = expected (labeled)
*0–30 days
†according to information given by LSOs
‡associated: a reasonable possibility of a causal relationship

Table 6 Requirements for foreign adverse event reports from clinical observational monitoring projects (COMP)*—All countries

Country	Time frame	Category	Causality
Argentina	none	none	
Bangladesh	none	none	
Belgium	none	none	
Brazil	none	none	
Chile	?	?	
Columbia	none	none	
Egypt	regulations under discussion		
Equador	no clear regulations		
Ghana	none	none	
Greece	none	none	
Guatemala	none	none	
Hong Kong	none	none	
India	none	none	
Indonesia	none	none	
Israel	none	none	
Italy	none	none	
Japan	none	none	
Korea	no time frame	ns/u, e	associated[†]
	no time frame	s/u, e	associated
Malaysia	none	none	
Mexico	none	none	
Nigeria	without time frame	ns/u, e	
	without time frame	s/u, e	
Peru	?	?	
Philippines	none	none	
Portugal	under discussion	?	
Singapore	?	?	
South Africa	none	none	
Sri Lanka	none	none	
Sweden	?	?	
Taiwan	none	none	
Thailand	none	none	
Turkey	none	none	
Uruguay	none	none	
Zimbabwe	none	none	

ns = non serious, s = serious, u = unexpected, e = expected
*according to information given by LSOs
[†]associated: a reasonable possibility of a causal relationship

A similar approach was taken in 1992 by Arnold Gordon (Gordon AJ, Petrick RJ, Drug Information Journal 1992; 26: 1–15). The results of both reports are somewhat different, which might be due to changes that occurred meanwhile in the requirements as well as different interpretation by local authorities and company members.

Concerning EC regulation, two different reporting systems are to be established, depending on the registration status of the drug. Final decisions and guidelines are expected soon.

17 Pharmacovigilance in the European Union

Gaby Danan

Rules and regulations

As of 1 January 1995, the European Union (EU) will have its pharmacovigilance regulations, i.e. a set of legal requirements regarding the monitoring of marketed drugs. Indeed, at present there is neither reporting obligation nor centralization of drug safety data at the European level. However, a system has existed for several years for the exchange of information between member states either regularly or in the event of a drug safety issue (the rapid alert system). This procedure allows problems to be raised and should theoretically avoid different decisions in the 12 countries of the EU concerning measures to be taken for public health. The drug company is informed either by one of the competent authorities in the EU or by a central body in Brussels. The pharmaceutical firm is allowed to defend its opinion during a session of the Pharmacovigilance Working Party, consisting of experts in drug safety from the member states and/or of the Committee for Proprietary Medicinal Products (CPMP). As the CPMP decisions are not binding on member states, different measures have been taken in the past for the same product: for example, aspirin and Reye's Syndrome; triazolam and psychiatric disorders.

The new regulations are now published in the Official Journal of the European Communities. They consist of two texts: a Council Regulation (1) and a Council Directive (2). The Council Regulation deals with the registration and monitoring of medicinal products according to the centralized procedure, implying the establishment of a new regulatory body: the European Agency for the Evaluation of Medicinal Products. The headquarters of this Agency will be located in London. Since it is a Council Regulation, the member states must apply all the provisions as soon as the Agency is ready to work i.e. as of 1 January 1995.

The Council Directive contains a chapter devoted to pharmacovigilance, providing the rules to be followed when drugs are registered according to the decentralized procedure.

This directive should enter in the regulations of member states on 1 January 1995 at the latest. As a Directive it only completes the legal obligations of pharmacovigilance that already exist in each member state.

Adverse Drug Reactions. A Practical Guide to Diagnosis and Management. Edited by C. Bénichou.
©1994 John Wiley & Sons Ltd.

In addition, it is clearly stated that the progress of international harmonization such as that made by ICH (International Conference for Harmonization) or CIOMS (Council for International Organizations of Medical Sciences) working parties will be taken into consideration by the European authorities.

Both regulation and directive, are accompanied by a set of at least five guidelines issued by the Pharmacovigilance working party in order to clarify or to complete some revisions. These guidelines should be published before end 1994.

For sake of clarity the presentation of the main regulatory requirements here will include first the definitions provided by the European authorities of the basic terms used in pharmacovigilance, then the obligations of the four parties involved: drug company, member states, Agency and Commission. Finally, the procedure followed in case of a drug safety issue will be briefly described.

Definitions of the basic terms used in pharmacovigilance

The article of the Council Directive dealing with the definitions is reproduced hereunder:

- "adverse reaction" means a reaction which is harmful and unintended and which occurs at doses normally used in man for the prophylaxis, diagnosis or treatment of disease or the modification of physiological function,
- "serious adverse reaction" means an adverse reaction which is fatal, life-threatening, disabling, incapacitating, or which results in or prolongs hospitalization,
- "unexpected adverse reaction" means an adverse reaction which is not mentioned in the summary of product characteristics,
- "serious unexpected adverse reaction" means an adverse reaction which is both serious and unexpected.

What are the obligations of the parties?

Whatever the registration procedure the obligations are identical except for the fact that the drug company has no direct link with the Agency when the drug has been registered according to the decentralized procedure. Other minor discrepancies will be indicated if necessary.

Obligations of the drug company

1. The person responsible for placing a medicinal product on the market *must be located* in the Community.

2. A qualified person responsible for pharmacovigilance is required *permanently and continuously* and shall be at the disposal of the person responsible for placing a medicinal product on the market.
   What are the main tasks of this qualified person?

   - Establishment and maintenance of a system that ensures collection, evaluation and collation of all adverse drug reactions (ADRs) reported by health care professionals to any employee of the company. The data shall be accessible at *a single point within the EU.*
   - Preparation of periodic reports.
   - Full and prompt answers to any request regarding the evaluation of benefits and risks and the volume of sales and prescriptions for the medicinal product concerned.

3. To maintain detailed records of all ADRs.

4. To inform member states and the Agency of serious and/or unexpected ADRs as indicated in Figure 1 when the drug has been registered according to the centralized procedure and as indicated in Figure 2 when the decentralized procedure has been applied.

As shown in Figure 1, *serious* ADRs are transmitted only to countries where they have occurred, while *serious* and *unexpected* ADRs should be transmitted to all member states and to the Agency.

As shown in Figure 2, all serious ADRs should be sent to the competent authority, which may be interpreted as the authority of the country in which the effect has occurred, provided the drug is sold in that country.

The time interval of 15 days begins on the day when an employee of the company and particularly a medical representative first receives information on the ADR.

Concerning the minimal information and the format of the report, the texts published do not give the details but it would seem probable that they will not be very different from those proposed by the CIOMS I Working Group.

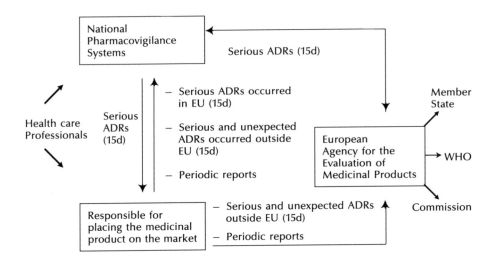

Figure 1 Pharmacovigilance reporting in the European Union. Centralized Procedure

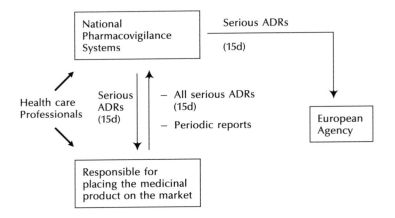

Figure 2 Pharmacovigilance reporting in the European Union. Decentralized Procedure

5. To submit a periodic report containing all records of ADRs and scientific evaluation every 6 months during the first 2 years, then once a year for the following 3 years then every 5 years together with the application of renewal of the authorization, or

- immediately upon request, or
- in case of a special requirement laid down as a condition of the granting of authorization.

The contents and format of this report are not yet indicated by the official text but they will probably be similar to those proposed by the CIOMS II Working Group. Some European countries already accept this type of report and a few members of the competent authorities of the EU participated in this Working Group.

6. To inform forthwith the Agency, the Commission and the member states of any prohibition or restriction imposed by any country or any new information that might influence the evaluation of the benefits and risks of its medicinal product. This includes any new information drawn from experimental or human studies or administrative measures.

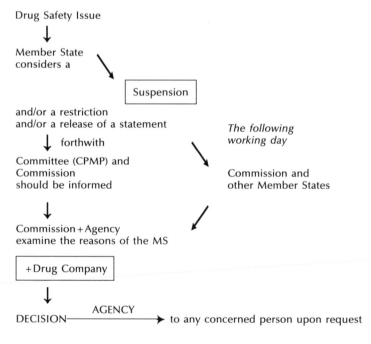

Figure 3 Procedure in the case of a drug safety issue

Obligations of the member states

1. To encourage health care professionals to report suspected ADRs to the authorities.
2. To report to the Agency and the drug company any serious ADR which occurred in its territory within 15 days following the receipt of the information. This obligation is new. It assures a real exchange of information between the drug company and the authorities.

Obligations of the Agency

1. To set up a data-processing network for the rapid transmission of information related to faulty manufacture, serious ADRs and other pharmacovigilance data.
2. To collaborate with the WHO on international pharmacovigilance and to inform this organization of the measures taken in the Community.

Obligation of the Commission

To draw up guidance on the collection, verification and presentation of ADRs.

Summarized procedure in the case of a drug safety issue

The current procedure called the "rapid alert system" is triggered when a member state is faced with a serious problem associated with the use of a drug. This procedure will be maintained in the future. In this case, the use of the product within the state boundaries can be suspended, but the state must inform the Agency and the other member states by the following working day, at the latest.

Figure 3 is a flow chart of the procedure in the case of a drug safety issue.

Conclusion

The European Agency is therefore confirmed as a new entity involved in drug safety evaluation with drug companies, and particularly for products that have been registered according to the centralized procedure.

To sum up, companies who want to market a drug in the European Union and to comply with the new regulations, should have an office in one of the EU countries where all information concerning the drug is available and at the disposal of a qualified person responsible for pharmacovigilance.

References

(1) Council Regulation (EEC) No. 2309/93 of 22 July 1993. Official Journal of the European Communities, 1993, L214 (24.8.93), 1–21.

(2) Council Directive 93/39/EEC of 14 June 1993. Official Journal of the European Communities, 1993, L 214 (24.8.93), 22–30.

18 Harmonization of international reporting of safety information for marketed drugs: the proposals of the CIOMS Working Groups I and II

Christian Bénichou

Drug regulatory agencies and pharmaceutical manufacturers have the task of making the use of medicines as effective and safe as possible. To do so, available international information must be consistently and appropriately analyzed and reported before and after approval.

Post-marketing surveillance is critical to ensuring the safety of approved drugs since clinical trials cannot be large enough, be of sufficient duration or involve enough subsets of patients to be able to detect rare side effects or drug interactions. In recognition of the global marketing of pharmaceutical products, regulators have increasingly required manufacturers to obtain and collect postapproval information from other countries. However, countries differ in their requirements and different authorities request that information from the same source be presented according to different inclusion criteria, formats and time intervals.

CIOMS* provided a forum for manufacturers and regulators to work together and test standard procedures regarding expedited (individual cases) and periodic (updated) reporting. Between 1986 and 1989 the Working Group on International Reporting of Adverse Drug Reactions (now called the CIOMS Working Group I) developed a uniform approach and format for reporting suspected adverse drug reactions (ADRs) occurring in foreign countries. The group was composed of members of six regulatory agencies and seven

---

*The CIOMS (Council for International Organizations of Medical Sciences) is an international, nongovernmental, nonprofit organization established in 1949 under the auspices of the WHO (World Health Organization) and the United Nations Educational, Scientific and Cultural Organization (UNESCO).

Adverse Drug Reactions. A Practical Guide to Diagnosis and Management. Edited by C. Bénichou.
©1994 John Wiley & Sons Ltd.

pharmaceutical manufacturers. In November 1989, a reconvened ADR working group (CIOMS Working Group II), consisting of members of the first group and others invited from industry and regulatory authorities, met to explore the possibility of developing harmonized or standardized approaches to safety update summaries including both domestic and foreign sources. A safety update by its nature is not an alert; rather, it should provide a review of information accumulated from various sources since the previous report, put into context against previous information.

Working Groups I and II could only make proposals, which can be summarized as presented in the following pages.

International expedited reporting of individual adverse drug reactions†

CIOMS reports are reports that include a minimum standard of information, submitted by manufacturers to regulatory bodies on the prescribed **CIOMS form**, concerning **serious, unlabelled adverse reactions** to **marketed drugs**, occurring in patients in **foreign countries**.

The CIOMS Working Group I developed the single form and set of definitions, procedures and methods and tested them in a pilot project demonstrating the feasibility and utility of a standard method.

All terms for procedures need to be defined:

1. Minimum standard of information

Four items constitute this minimum: an identifiable source, a patient (even if not precisely identified by name and date of birth), a suspect drug and a suspect reaction.

2. CIOMS form

The format for reporting called the CIOMS form is presented in Figures 1a and 1b (see explanatory notes on completion of the CIOMS form on page 256).

3. A reaction

This is to be distinguished from an event since a reaction implies that a professional health care worker has judged it a reasonable possibility that an observed clinical occurrence was caused by a drug.

4. Serious

A serious reaction is a reaction that is fatal or life-threatening, or has involved or prolonged inpatient hospitalization, or resulted in persistent or significant disability or incapacity.

5. Unlabelled

A reaction is unlabelled when it is not mentioned in the approved information on the drug in the country of reporting.

---

†International Reporting of Adverse Drug Reactions, Final Report of CIOMS Working Group, Geneva, 1990.

SUSPECT ADVERSE REACTION REPORT

1. REACTION INFORMATION

1. PATIENT INITIALS (first, last)	1a. COUNTRY	2. DATE OF BIRTH			2a. AGE Years	3. SEX	4-6. REACTION ONSET			8-12. CHECK ALL APPROPRIATE TO ADVERSE REACTION
		Day	Month	Year			Day	Month	Year	

7 + 13. DESCRIBE REACTION(S) (including relevant tests/lab data)

8-12. CHECK ALL APPROPRIATE TO ADVERSE REACTION

☐ PATIENT DIED

☐ INVOLVED OR PROLONGED INPATIENT HOSPITALIZATION

☐ INVOLVED PERSISTENCE OR SIGNIFICANT DISABILITY OR INCAPACITY

☐ LIFE THREATENING

II. SUSPECT DRUG(S) INFORMATION

14. SUSPECT DRUG(S) (include generic name)

15. DAILY DOSE(S)

16. ROUTE(S) OF ADMINISTRATION

17. INDICATION(S) FOR USE

18. THERAPY DATES (from/to)

19. THERAPY DURATION

20. DID REACTION ABATE AFTER STOPPING DRUG?
☐ YES   ☐ NO   ☐ NA

21. DID REACTION REAPPEAR AFTER REINTRODUCTION?
☐ YES   ☐ NO   ☐ NA

III. CONCOMITANT DRUG(S) AND HISTORY

22. CONCOMITANT DRUG(S) AND DATES OF ADMINISTRATION (exclude those used to treat reaction)
23. OTHER RELEVANT HISTORY (e.g. diagnostics, allergics, pregnancy with last month of period, etc.)

IV. MANUFACTURER INFORMATION

24a. NAME AND ADDRESS OF MANUFACTURER	24b. MFR CONTROL NO.
	24d. REPORT SOURCE □ STUDY □ LITERATURE □ HEALTH PROFESSIONAL
24c. DATE RECEIVED BY MANUFACTURER	25a. REPORT TYPE □ INITIAL □ FOLLOWUP
DATE OF THIS REPORT	

Figure 1a The CIOMS form

1. Country of origin of report (item 1a). It was suggested that the WHO list of abbreviations could be used but that the country name be written out wherever there is the possibility of error.

2. Hospitalization (item 9). Used when the reaction resulted in, was directly associated with, or prolonged hospitalization. Does not mean only that the ADR happened to occur in a hospitalized patient.

3. Definition of "life-threatening" (item 12). Most members of the group felt this was self-evident. Generally, this refers to the imminent and markedly increased likelihood of death.

4. Description of the reaction (item 13). Use an English translation of the language in which the reaction was originally reported.

5. Suspect and concomitant drugs (items 14 and 22). Give the generic name of the main active ingredient (regardless of salt and dose) and of the other active ingredients. The WHO Drug Reference List provides valuable information for assisting with this. (18)

6. In the US, in contrast to the rest of the world, dates are expressed numerically in the sequence of month, day and year. Consequently, for international usage the dates on the report must include the abbreviated name of the month, e.g. JAN 4 or 4 JAN, rather than 0104.

7. In the US forms must be designated as 15-Day forms. This may be done by rubber-stamping forms submitted to the FDA.

8. The CIOMS form should be submitted in English.

9. As to the legal status of the form, it should be viewed as a recommended prototype subject to modification by manufacturers who choose to use it or by regulatory authorities who choose to accept it. In every instance, manufacturers who use the form should clear such use with the receiving regulatory authorities.

Figure 1b Explanatory notes on completion of the CIOMS form

6. Time of reporting

Manufacturers should submit completed CIOMS report forms to regulatory authorities as soon as they are received, and in no case later than 15 working days after their receipt. The 15-day period begins as soon as a company, or any part or affiliate of a company, receives the report. Manufacturers must therefore continue to seek to accelerate communications between themselves and their affiliates.

International reporting of periodic drug safety update summaries[‡]

Some additional definitions are needed

1. Core data sheet (international prescribing information)

A document prepared by the pharmaceutical manufacturer, containing all relevant safety information, such as adverse drug reactions, which the manufacturer stipulates should be listed for the drug in all countries where the drug is marketed. It is the international reference document by which "labelled" and "unlabelled" are determined, which differs from the above definitions of labelling for the CIOMS Working Group I reports.

2. Data lock-point (cut-off date)

The date designated as the cut-off date for data to be incorporated into a particular safety update. On this date the data available to the author of the safety report are extracted for review and stored.

3. International birth date

The date on which the first regulatory authority approved a particular drug for marketing. The proposal is that the manufacturer's data are extracted for review of the particular drug every 6 months subsequently, and that all regulatory authorities that wish to have safety updates will accept the same cut-off date.

4. Serious

In addition to the four categories specified on the CIOMS form designed by the CIOMS Working Group I, CIOMS safety updates require consideration of all drug interactions, cases of drug abuse, and cases of significant overdosage; therefore these cases could also be considered "serious" and included in line listings in CIOMS safety updates or added as a separate table.

Scope

1. Subject drugs for review

The proposal was that summary updates in the proposed format should be prepared for all new chemical entities licensed for the first time during 1992 and thereafter subsequent updates would include data for a specified 6-month review period.

[‡]International Reporting of Periodic Drug-Safety Update Summaries, Final Report of CIOMS Working Group II, Geneva 1992.

2. Frequency of review

Each subject drug will have an international birth date, which will be the date on which the first regulatory authority approved the drug. The manufacturer's database will be frozen for each particular drug every 6 months subsequently.

The implication of this is that, irrespective of date of approval, all regulators requesting or expecting to receive CIOMS periodic reports will receive them within the first 6 months of the drug's approval in their countries, and then subsequently at 6-monthly intervals. Normally the manufacturer would make each report available within 45 calendar days of the data lock-point.

Content

See Figure 2.

PERIODIC SAFETY UPDATE SUMMARY
(CIOMS Working Group II)

I—INTRODUCTION

– Presentation of the drug
– Presentation of the report
   "Reference should be made to not only product(s) covered by the report but also those excluded because, for example, they are covered in another manufacturer's or in a separate moiety report. Data from co-marketers or licensees should be included unless it is known that they are submitting their own safety updates."

II—CORE DATA SHEET

Basic product information containing all relevant safety information to be mentioned in all countries except locally required addition or deletion. It is the reference document by which "labelled" and "unlabelled" are determined.

III—DRUG'S LICENSED STATUS FOR MARKETING (the only section that is cumulative)

List of dates and countries in which a regulatory (or voluntary) decision has been taken (approved, approved with qualification, rejected, etc.) for safety reasons.

Dates of approval (or rejection) and of market introduction.

Trade names in different countries.

IV—UPDATE OF REGULATORY OR MANUFACTURER ACTIONS TAKEN FOR SAFETY REASONS

– Suspension, restriction to distribution, any curtailment of trial programmes, significant alterations to label/package insert
– Format: brief narrative stating the reasons with appended documentation.

V—PATIENT EXPOSURE

– As number of prescriptions, or tonnage, or patient-days exposure.

VI—INDIVIDUAL CASE HISTORIES

Sources:
a) relevant individual case reports from studies (published or unpublished): serious, unlabelled, and attributable to the drug
b) spontaneous reports: serious or unlabelled
c) published individual case histories: all serious, or unexpected non serious
d) serious case reports from other sources (regulatory authorities, other manufacturers); be comprehensive but avoid duplication of reporting.

Format:
– presented in body system order
– in the format of a CIOMS line listing (see Figure 3)
– when necessary, include a brief narrative based on the manufacturer's analysis, including a comment on increase of frequency.

VII—STUDIES

– Newly analyzed studies containing *important* safety information.
– Targeted new safety studies (either initiated during the period of review or continuing)
– Published safety studies, new important safety findings (positive or negative) found on review of published toxicological, clinical and epidemiological studies.

continued

Figure 2 Periodic safety update summary (CIOMS Working Group II)

continued ─────────────────────────────────────

VIII—OVERALL SAFETY EVALUATION

- Concise critical analysis and opinion on increased frequency of known toxicity
- Drug interactions
- Overdose and its treatment
- Drug abuse
- Positive and negative experiences during pregnancy or lactation
- Effects of long-term treatment
- Any specific safety issues relating to special patient groups, such as the elderly or the very young.

IX—IMPORTANT INFORMATION RECEIVED AFTER DATA LOCK-POINT
New cases on follow-up data that affect the interpretation or evaluation of existing reports.

Figure 2   Continued

Presented in body system order for the most serious presenting sign or symptom:

COLUMNS:

Country

Source, e.g. trialist, physician, literature

Age

Sex

Dose of the drug

Duration of treatment (prior to event); time to onset

Description of reaction (as reported)

Outcome, e.g. fatal, resolved

(Comment)

Company reference number

Figure 3   CIOMS Standardized Line Listing of Adverse Drug Reactions*

Summaries should include combination products, with reference to the active moiety. It will often be appropriate in a given report to separate different formulations, routes of administration, and indications (if this information is available).

When relevant, the safety update could also differentiate data associated with salient pharmaceutical facts, including the active moiety or moieties, excipients, strength(s) and dosage form(s), etc.

───

*WHO codes could be used for some items.

19 WHO adverse drug reactions terminology: from terminology to dictionary

Ralph Edwards, Gaby Danan, Cecilia Biriell and Christian Bénichou

During an International Consensus Meeting on Drug-Induced Liver Disorders, held in Paris in June 1989, under the auspices of the Council of International Organizations of Medical Sciences (CIOMS) the participants were asked for a list of clinical or laboratory abnormalities of the liver or biliary tract that could be drug-induced, which were then defined (J Hepatol 1990; 11: 272–6.). As a pilot project, the WHO Collaborating Centre for International Drug Monitoring in Uppsala, Sweden, in collaboration with the organizers of the meeting, proposed a revised version of section 0700 (Liver and Biliary Tract Disorders) of WHO-ART (WHO Adverse Drug Reaction Terminology) along the lines of the recommendations of the Consensus Meeting.

The extension of these recommendations as part of the WHO-ART hierachical terminology improves its precision and its adaptation to evolving investigative procedures and to the description of hepatic or biliary lesions likely to be drug-induced.

The use of definitions and guidelines may aid all those reporting and analyzing suspected drug adverse reactions. More consistent use of these recognized terms, however, does not preclude the use of other descriptions of hepatic adverse drug reactions if necessary, nor does it imply that reports which do not use the terms completely as defined are of less public health import. It should be possible to "flag" reports that meet the definitions, or to use the designation "not otherwise specified" (NOS), as we have done for some terms in Table 1.

The revision of the WHO-ART is based on:

1. The addition of new terms corresponding to definitions that are widely accepted or drawn from the conclusions of the Consensus Meeting;

Adverse Drug Reactions. A Practical Guide to Diagnosis and Management. Edited by C. Bénichou.
©1994 John Wiley & Sons Ltd.

2. The definitions of existing terms;
3. Recommendations for the use of all the terms that have been used for reporting of ADRs in the section. Certain terms have been identified that should not be used unless they correspond to histologic lesions, which makes a liver biopsy necessary.

As a general rule, the "Preferred Terms" should have priority in the designation of disorders. The expression "High Level Term" has been dropped and replaced by the more explicit expression "Grouping Terms". These grouping terms are primarily intended to aid search strategies and should not be used for reporting since they are not precise; exceptionally they can be useful when information is insufficient. Finally, there are the "Included Terms," which are near-synonyms for the "Preferred Terms" or "Grouping Terms" generally used by the reporters.

Table 1 System Organ Class: Liver and biliary tract disorders 0700

Definitions of preferred terms or Recommendations for use	Preferred terms / *Included terms to preferred*	Grouping terms / *Included terms to group*
Requires cholangiography	Bile duct stricture	Biliary tract disorder
Requires cholangiography	Biliary atresia	*Gall bladder disorder*
Usually, pain is localized in the epigastrium or the right hypochondrium, referred below the right scapula, rises acutely to a plateau, can last 30–60 minutes and is associated with abnormalities of the biliary tract confirmed by imaging	Biliary pain / *Biliary cholic* / *Spasm biliary*	
Ultrasonographic abnormality defined as mobile hyperechogenic material in the gall bladder (thick bile or gall bladder pseudolithiasis)	Biliary sludge	
Requires imaging or surgical or histological examination	Cholecystitis	
Requires imaging, ultrasonography or cholangiography	Cholelithiasis / *Gall bladder stones* / *Common bile duct stones*	
Requires liver histology	Hepatic cirrhosis	Cirrhosis
Cirrhosis caused by intrahepatic as well as extrahepatic bile duct diseases Requires liver histology	Cirrhosis biliary / *Pseudo primary biliary cirrhosis* / *Secondary biliary cirrhosis*	
Listed in liver disorders as it can be a complication of portal hypertension (see this term)	Haematemesis / *Oesophageal haemorrhage* / *Gastric haemorrhage* / *Vomiting blood*	GI haemorrhage / Gastrointestinal tract bleed NOS
Listed in liver disorders as it can be a complication of portal hypertension (see this term)	Haemorrhage rectum / *Haematochezia* / *Faeces blood stained*	
Listed in liver disorders as it can be a complication of portal hypertension (see this term)	Melaena / *Stool tarry* / *Stool black*	

continued overleaf

Table 1 (continued)

Definitions of preferred terms or Recommendations for use	Preferred terms / Included terms to preferred	Grouping terms / Included terms to group
Combination of hepatic encephalopathy and severe coagulation disorders	Hepatic failure acute	Hepatic failure
Rapid development (days or weeks) of hepatic encephalopathy after the onset of jaundice	Hepatic failure fulminant Fulminant hepatitis	
Designates acute prerenal failure complicating severe acute or chronic liver disease; to be distinguished from combined acute renal and liver failure	Hepatorenal syndrome	
Increase of alkaline phosphatase whatever the figure over N	Alkaline phosphatase increased	Hepatic function abnormal Hepatic dysfunction nonicteric
Figures should be provided	Alpha-fetoprotein increased	AG ratio abnormal
Describe the abnormality	BSP test abnormal Bromsulphthalein retention Sulphobromophthalein retention	Albumin globulin ratio abnormal Cephalin flocculation abnormal
Increase in GGT whatever the figures over N	Gamma-GT increased Gamma-glutamyltransferase incr. GT elevated GT increased	CFT abnormal Liver function tests abnormal NOS Liver tests abnormality NOS Thymol turbidity abnormal
Increase in AST whatever the figures over N	AST increased Glutamic-oxaloacetic transam. inc Serum glutamic-oxaloacetic ta inc SGOT increased	
If figures below 2 times the upper limit of normal	ALT increased Glutamic-pyruvic transam. inc Serum glutamic-pyruvic transam inc SGPT increased	
	Hepatorenal syndrome	
Figures below 50% of control	Proaccelerin (factor V) decreased	
Focal necrosis due to local ischaemia within the liver	Hepatic infarction	Hepatic necrosis

Description	Term	Higher-level term
Designates acute hepatocellular liver injury due to hypoxaemia or sudden fall of hepatic blood flow	Hepatic necrosis, ischaemic	
Liver histology is required	Hepatic neoplasm benign	Hepatic neoplasm NOS
Liver histology is required	Hepatic neoplasm malignant	Hepatic tumor
Liver histology is required	Hepatitis acute	Hepatitis
Liver histology is required	Hepatitis chronic active	Hepatitis toxic
Liver histology is required	Hepatitis chronic	Hepatitis NOS
Liver histology is required	Hepatitis chronic persistent	Hepatitis granulomatous Liver tender
Requires liver histology (demonstrating impairment of the formation and/or flow of bile). Otherwise, should be replaced by 'liver injury cholestatic' or 'liver test abnormality'	Hepatitis cholestatic *Cholangiolitis toxic* *Cholestasis intrahepatic* *Hepatitis toxic obstructive* Chronic cholestatic syndrome	Hepatitis
Requires liver histology and/or microbiologic procedures and/or serologic markers	Hepatitis viral	Hepatitis infectious
Requires liver histology and/or microbiologic procedures and/or serologic markers	Hepatitis bacterial	
Requires liver histology and/or microbiologic procedures and/or serologic markers	Hepatitis mycotic	
Requires liver histology and microbiologic procedures	Hepatitis parasitic	
Should be used when: • histological data are not available • and if there is an increase; − over 2N (N is the upper limit of normal range) in alanine aminotransferase (ALT) or in conjugated bilirubin, or combined increase in aspartate aminotransferase (AST), alkaline phosphatase (AP) and total bilirubin (TB) provided one of them is over 2N	Liver injury acute	Liver injury *Hepatic damage* *Hepatic disease* *Hepatotoxic effect*

continued overleaf

Table 1 *(continued)*

Definitions of preferred terms or Recommendations for use	Preferred terms / *Included terms to preferred*	Grouping terms / *Included terms to group*
• 'chronic' when these elevations have lasted more than 3 months (this should be distinguished from 'chronic liver disease', which may be used only on the basis of histological findings)	Liver injury chronic	Liver injury (cont'd)
According to the ratio (R) ALT/AP, where each activity is expressed as a multiple of N (both activities should be measured at the time of recognition of liver injury)	Liver injury hepatocellular / *Liver cell damage* / *Hepatocellular damage*	
• 'hepatocellular' when there is an increase of over 2N in ALT alone or R>5		
• 'acute' when the increases have lasted less than 3 months	Liver injury hepatocellular acute	
• 'chronic' when the increases have lasted more than 3 months (this should be distinguished from 'chronic liver disease', which may be used only on the basis of histological findings)	Liver injury hepatocellular chronic	
• 'cholestatic' when there is an increase over 2N in AP alone or R≤2	Liver injury cholestatic	
• 'acute' when the increases have lasted less than 3 months	Liver injury cholestatic acute	
• 'chronic' when the increases have lasted more than 3 months (this should be distinguished from 'chronic liver disease', which may be used only on the basis of histological findings)	Liver injury cholestatic chronic	
• 'mixed' when both ALT (above 2N) and AP are increased, and 2<R<5	Liver injury mixed	

Liver injury (cont'd)	Liver injury mixed acute	• 'acute' when the increases have lasted less than 3 months
	Liver injury mixed chronic	• 'chronic' when the increases have lasted more than 3 months (this should be distinguished from 'chronic liver disease', which may be used only on the basis of histological findings)
Liver fatty *Liver fatty deposition* *Liver fatty infiltration* *Liver fatty metamorphosis* *Liver fatty phanerosis* *Liver fatty change* *Liver fatty degeneration*	Liver fatty macrovesicular	Requires liver histology to distinguish from the microvesicular type
	Liver fatty microvesicular	Requires liver histology to distinguish from the macrovesicular type
Jaundice	Bilirubin total increased *Biliverdin increased* *Hyperbilirubinaemia* *Bilirubinaemia* *Bilirubin increased*	Figures of total bilirubin over the upper limit of normal range
	Bilirubinaemia conjugated increased	
	Bilirubinuria *Choluria* Bilirubinaemia aggravated	When figures are between N and 2N
—	Ascites	Presence of liquid in the peritoneal cavity
—	Bile duct carcinoma *Gall bladder carcinoma* *Carcinoma bile duct*	Requires histological evidence

continued overleaf

Table 1 *(continued)*

Definitions of preferred terms or Recommendations for use	Preferred terms *Included terms to preferred*	Grouping terms *Included terms to group*
Requires imaging and/or histology demonstrating obstruction of intra-hepatic binding tree	Cholangitis toxic	—
idem	Cholangiolitis toxic	—
Should be associated with a specific sign of liver disorder	Faeces clay-coloured *Faeces discoloured* *Faeces pale*	—
Liver histology is required	Granulomatous liver disease	—
To be used only when associated with cirrhosis Otherwise should be coded in the section 1410	Gynaecomastia *Breast enlargement male*	—
Disturbances of central nervous system associated with hepatic failure, generally flapping tremor asterixis) and/or disturbed consciousness, then coma in severe cases	Hepatic encephalopathy *Coma hepatic*	—
Requires liver histology	Hepatic fibrosis	—
Requires liver histology	Hepatic haemorrhage	—
Requires imaging or histological evidence	Hepatic vein thrombosis *Budd-Chiari syndrome*	—
Liver histology is required	Hepatitis neonatal *Hepatocellular damage neonatal*	—
Needs confirmation by ultrasonography of the increase in the size of the liver	Hepatomegaly *Liver enlargement*	—
Needs confirmation by ultrasonography of the increase in the size of the spleen and of the liver	Hepatosplenomegaly	—
Needs confirmation by ultrasonography of the increase in the size of the spleen and of the liver	Hepatosplenomegaly neonatal	—
Requires demonstration of increased pressure in the portal system, or of occlusion or obstruction of the portal vein, or of consequences of portal hypertension such as gastro-oesophageal varices or enlarged spleen or splenic vein	Hypertension portal	—

Needs confirmation of increased value of bilirubinaemia	Jaundice neonatal *Jaundice of newborn* *Bilirubinaemia newborn* *Icterus neonatorum*	—
Liver histology is required, demonstrating perinuclear deposits of eosinophilic material within the altered hepatocytes	Mallory's bodies	—
Liver histology is required, demonstrating blood filled cavities corresponding to dilatation of sinusoids	Peliosis hepatis	—
Liver histology is required, demonstrating accumulation of phospholipids	Phospholipidosis	—
Requires biochemical demonstration of overproduction of heme precursors	Porphyria *Porphyria type syndrome* *Porphyrins urinary excretion increased* *Uroporphyrin excretion increased*	—
Acute disease characterized by vomiting, hepatic encephalopathy and microvesicular fatty liver	Reye's syndrome	—
Requires imaging and/or histology, demonstrating obstruction of the extra- and intrahepatic biliary tree by fibroinflammatory tissue	Sclerosing cholangitis Cholangitis NOS	—
Liver histology is required	Sinusoidal dilatation	—
Requires liver histology, demonstrating obliteration of the centrilobular and sublobular hepatic veins	Veno-occlusive liver disease	—

20 Imputability of unexpected or toxic drug reactions

Christian Bénichou

The official French method of causality assessment

In France manufacturers of drugs that have received marketing authorization should declare to the Commission Nationale de Pharmacovigilance all the adverse reactions that have been reported to them. This "déclaration obligatoire" is done every 6 months during the first year of marketing and then once every year after that.

One of the characteristics of the French regulations is that the role of each drug be evaluated, using the official method of causality assessment, a revised version of which was published in 1985.* This method distinguishes between intrinsic imputability which takes into account only the information available on the case report to be assessed and an extrinsic imputability, based on all published data on all drugs. Intrinsic imputability is calculated independently for each drug taken but without taking into account the degree of imputability of the concomitant drugs.

---

*Moore N, Paux G, Begaud B, Biour M, Loupi E, Boismare F, Royer RJ, Advese Drug Reaction Monitoring: Doing it the French Way. Lancet; 1985 November: 1058.

Adverse Drug Reactions. A Practical Guide to Diagnosis and Management. Edited by C. Bénichou.
©1994 John Wiley & Sons Ltd.

Intrinsic imputability

Two groups of criteria, chronological and semeiological, are used.

Chronological criteria

There are three (see Table 1):

- The **time interval** separating administration of the drug and onset of the adverse reaction may be described as very suggestive, compatible or incompatible.
- The **course** of the reaction **when the drug is stopped** may be described as suggestive, inconclusive and nonsuggestive (that is, against the role of the drug).
- The results of **readministration** of the drug (which is generally accidental and involuntary since rarely without risks). Readministration can be evaluated as positive, $(R+)$, negative $(R-)$ or uninterpretable $(R0)$.

The combination of these three criteria results in an intermediate chronological score (C) with four possibilities: **C3** likely chronology, **C2** possible chronology, **C1** doubtful chronology and **C0** incompatible chronology (see Table 1).

Table 1   Chronological criteria

| | Time to onset | | | | | | |
| | very suggestive | | | compatible | | | |
Readministration	$(R+)$	$(R0)$	$R(-)$	$R(+)$	$R(0)$	$R(-)$	incompatible
Course							
— suggestive	C3	C3	C1	C3	C2	C1	C0
— inconclusive	C3	C2	C1	C3	C1	C1	C0
— not suggestive	C1	C1	C1	C1	C1	C1	C0

C0 = incompatible chronology   C2 = possible chronology
C1 = doubtful chronology   C3 = suggestive chronology

Semeiological criteria

These take into account (Table 2):

- "semeiology" itself, that is the clinical or paraclinical picture which may or may not be evocative of the role of the drug, as well as the existence of validated risk factors;
- the search for other causes which may have revealed that they are absent or remain possible;
- finally, for certain reactions, reliable and specific laboratory tests which may or may not have been performed with positive results.

Table 2 Semeiological criteria

| | SEMEIOLOGY | | | | | |
| | suggestive of the role of the drug or favorizing factors | | | other cases | | |
	L(+)	L(0)	L(−)	L(+)	L(0)	L(−)
SPECIFIC TEST						
Absent	S3	S3	S1	S3	S2	S1
NONDRUG CAUSE						
Possible	S3	S2	S1	S3	S1	S1
(or not searched for)						

S1 = doubtful semeiology   S2 = possible semeiology   S3 = suggestive semeiology   L = laboratory test

The combination of these different criteria (see Table 2) results in a score with three possibilities: **S3** suggestive semeiology, **S2** possible semeiology and **S1** doubtful semeiology.

Intrinsic imputability score

The combination of the two preceding decision tables results in a final assessment score (Table 3) with five possibilities ranging from I0 to I4; thus the roles of the drug appears as unlikely, doubtful, possible, likely or very likely.

Table 3 Final imputation

| | SEMIOLOGY | S1 | S2 | S3 |
CHRONOLOGY				
C0		I0	I0	I0
C1		I1	I1	I2
C2		I1	I2	I3
C3		I3	I3	I4

I0 = unlikely   I1 = doubtful   I2 = possible   I3 = likely   I4 = very likely

Extrinsic imputability: scoring of bibliographic data

Analysis of available published data results in a 4-degree score ranging from B0 to B3, indicating an increasing degree of previous knowledge of the evaluated reaction.

Published (bibliographic) data are also scored, as **B3** (when the side effect has been described in the standard textbooks), **B2** (when a similar effect has been described for the drug concerned or for a related drug, or when the effect can be expected from experimental data), **B0** (or when no relevant report can be found despite an extensive search through literature, including computerized databanks—this score is used only for a well-documented case, worthy of being published), or **B1** (none of the above).

Comments

A comment concerning reactions that occur after stopping the treatment: it would have been necessary to analyze—along with the usual time to onset, i.e. the interval separating the start of administration of a drug from the occurrence of the reaction another interval for some cases which is the time between the end of treatment and the appearance of the reaction. Additionally, the semeiological criteria should at times evaluate the course of the reaction when the treatment has not been stopped if a drug origin was not suspected or recognized, treatment was then continued and the evolution should be interpreted differently.

This method aims at maximum sensitivity to the detriment of specific: it is intended as a means of detection. Easy to apply, it allows rapid scoring of the available information, ruling out all the cases assessed as I0 where the role of the drug is ruled out and retaining the observations where imputability is more than 1. It is very useful to set off an alert. However, use of the method is not obligatory when an investigation is underway and more specific evaluations appear necessary.

As it is standardized and mandatory, this method has given a common language to the administration and the pharmaceutical industry. The privileged role of intrinsic imputability, setting aside the weights of concomitant drugs, allows the taking account of the first cases of toxicity of a drug which may at times appear as less suspect than the associated drugs, the toxicity of which is recognized.

21 A new method for drug causality assessment: RUCAM

Christian Bénichou and Gaby Danan

The Consensus Meetings organized on adverse drug reactions have been presented in the introduction. Based on their results for causality assessment criteria, a new method has been proposed, named RUCAM (Roussel Uclaf Causality Assessment Method).

As most of the experts involved in the Consensus Meetings were specialists in their medical field and not specialists in "causality assessment," they could be asked to propose the content and limits of various criteria, but not to determine their weight. To attain a global score, it was necessary to assign weights, independently from the medical experts. It was decided that, for each criterion, the widest scale could range from -3 to $+3$, the criterion being at the maximum quantified in 7 degrees $(-3, -2, -1, 0, +1, +2, +3)$, corresponding to the increasing probability of the role of the drug evaluated. The following ranges have been retained for the different criteria (figure 1):

Time to onset and course of the reaction:
These two criteria were attributed the widest range $(-3, +3)$. The role of the drug must be ruled out by an incompatible time to onset. For some reactions, e.g. acute liver injury, when the time interval is unknown, the case report can be considered as "insufficiently documented" to allow any causality assessment.

The score of risk factors for the occurrence of adverse reactions does not exceed 2 points.

Screening for other causes includes two parts: assessment of the role of concomitant therapies and screening for non drug-related causes:

a) **assessment of the role of concomitant therapies** takes into account both the time relationship and the previous knowledge of their toxicity for this type of reaction. Demonstration of the role of a concomitant drug, for example further positive rechallenge, reduces the score by -3; however, this does not completely exonerate the evaluated drug, particularly in view of a possible interaction.

Adverse Drug Reactions. A Practical Guide to Diagnosis and Management. Edited by C. Bénichou.
©1994 John Wiley & Sons Ltd.

b) **screening for non drug-related causes** is particularly important for reactions that are rarely drug-induced, i.e. where the role of drugs in the etiology is not preponderant. In these situations, e.g. acute liver injury, if the most common non drug-related causes have not been sought, the score should be reduced by -2; the evidence of a recent non drug cause reduces the score by -3. This etiological investigation cannot have the same *value* for reactions where drugs generally have a preponderant etiological role (e.g. toxic epidermal necrolysis (TEN) or fixed drug eruption). Accordingly, the *value* of the investigation for non drug causes has to be adapted and validated for each reaction. Globally, the search for other causes cannot reduce the role of the drug evaluated by more than 4 points (-2 for unsought non drug causes, and -2 for a concomitant medication known to be toxic and with a compatible or suggestive time to onset).

Concerning previous knowledge of the toxicity of the evaluated drug, a score consisting of 3 degrees is proposed, i.e. 0 when the reaction is completely unknown for the drug, $+1$ if such cases have been published but not integrated into the product information, and $+2$ when it appears in the product characteristics.

Confirmation of the reaction by either *in vivo* (positive rechallenge) or *in vitro* tests or assays was attributed the widest range (-3, $+3$).

Theoretically the range of the *global* score would be -9 to $+15$ (Figure 1). In practice, after assessment of several hundreds of case reports of various drug reactions, it is between -5 and $+13$. That means that all arguments for, or all arguments against the role of the drug were not encountered in a single case.

Regarding the significance of these figures and their equivalence with the usual classifications, and for acute hepatic injuries, scores may be classified in 5 degrees: score $\leqslant 0$, relationship *"excluded"*; 1 to 2: *"unlikely"*; 3 to 5: *"possible"*; 6 to 8: *"probable"*; above 8: *"highly probable."*

Criteria	Score
1. TIME TO ONSET OF THE REACTION	
Highly suggestive	+3
Suggestive	+2
Compatible	+1
Inconclusive	0
If incompatible, then case "unrelated"	
If information not available, then case "insufficiently documented"	
2. COURSE OF THE REACTION	
Highly suggestive	+3
Suggestive	+2
Compatible	+1
Against the role of the drug	−2
Inconclusive or not available	0
3. RISK FACTOR(S) FOR DRUG REACTION	
Presence	+1[a]
Absence	0
4. CONCOMITANT DRUG(S)	
Time to onset incompatible	0
Time to onset compatible but unknown reaction	−1
Time to onset compatible and known reaction	−2
Role proved in this case	−3
None or information not available	0
5. NON-DRUG-RELATED CAUSES	
Ruled out	+2
Possible or not investigated[b]	+1 to −2
Probable	−3
6. PREVIOUS INFORMATION ON THE DRUG	
Reaction unknown	0
Reaction published but unlabelled	+1
Reaction labelled in the product characteristics	+2
7. RESPONSE TO READMINISTRATION	
Positive	+3
Compatible	+1
Negative	−2
Not available or not interpretable	0
or PLASMA CONCENTRATION of the drug known to be toxic	+3
or VALIDATED LABORATORY TEST with high specificity, sensitivity and predictive values	
Positive	+3
Negative	−3
Not interpretable or not available	0

[a] one additional point for every validated risk factor
[b] depending on the nature of the reaction

Figure 1 Method for causality assessment of adverse drug reactions (RUCAM)

DRUG └────────────────────────

CASE NO. └─┘└─┘/└─┘

REACTION ONSET └─┘/└─┘/└─┘

CAUSALITY ASSESSMENT OF A DRUG IN A CASE OF ACUTE LIVER INJURY

FORM COMPLETED ON └─┘/└─┘/└─┘

	HEPATOCELLULAR TYPE	CHOLESTATIC OR MIXED TYPE	ASSESSMENT
1. TIME TO ONSET			
Incompatible	Reaction occurred before starting the drug or more than 15 days after stopping the drug (except for slowly metabolized drugs)	Reaction occurred before starting the drug or more than 30 days after stopping the drug (except for slowly metabolized drugs)	UNRELATED
Unknown	When information is not available to calculate time to onset, then the case is		Insuff. documented

	INITIAL TREATMENT	SUBSEQUENT TREATMENT	INITIAL TREATMENT	SUBSEQUENT TREATMENT	SCORE (CIRCLE THE RESULTS)

—From the beginning of the drug
  Suggestive
  Compatible
	5–90 days
	<5 or >90 days
		1 to 15 days
		>15 days
			5 to 90 days
			<5 or >90 days
				1 to 90 days
				>90 days
					+2
					+1

—From cessation of the drug Compatible	≤15 days	≤15 days	≤30 days	≤30 days	+1

	HEPATOCELLULAR TYPE	CHOLESTATIC OR MIXED TYPE	SCORE
2. COURSE	DIFFERENCE BETWEEN THE PEAK OF ALT (SGPT) AND UPPER LIMIT OF NORMAL VALUES	DIFFERENCE BETWEEN THE PEAK OF AP (or TB) AND UPPER LIMIT OF NORMAL VALUES	

After cessation of the drug
  Highly suggestive
  Suggestive
  Compatible
  Inconclusive
	Decrease ≥50% within 8 days
	Decrease ≥50% within 30 days
	Not applicable
	No information or
		Not applicable
		Decrease ≥50% within 180 days
		Decrease <50% within 180 days
		Persistence or increase or no information
			+3
			+2
			+1
			0

Against the role of the drug	Decrease ≥50%, after the 30th day Decrease <50%, after the 30th day	No situation	0
If the drug is continued Inconclusive	or recurrent increase All situations	*Not applicable* All situations	−2 0

Figure 2 Criteria for drug-induced liver injuries

	Ethanol	Ethanol or Pregnancy	
3. RISK FACTORS			
Presence			+1
Absence			0
Age of the patient ≥55 years			+1
Age of the patient <55 years			0
4. CONCOMITANT DRUG(S)			
None or no information or concomitant drugs with incompatible time to onset			0
Concomitant drug with compatible or suggestive time to onset			−1
Concomitant drug known as hepatotoxin and with compatible or suggestive time to onset			−2
Concomitant drug with evidence for its role in this case (positive rechallenge or validated test)			−3
5. SEARCH FOR NONDRUG CAUSES			
Group I (6 causes)= RECENT VIRAL INFECTION WITH HAV (IgM anti-HAV antibody) or HBV (IgM anti-HBc antibody) or HCV (anti-HCV antibody and circumstantial arguments for non A—non B hepatitis); BILIARY OBSTRUCTION (ultrasonography); ALCOHOLISM (AST/ALT ≥2); ACUTE RECENT HYPOTENSION HISTORY (particularly if underlying heart disease) Group II= Complications of underlying disease(s); Clinical and/or biological context suggesting CMV, EBV or Herpes virus infection		• All causes—groups I and II—reasonably ruled out	+2
		• The 6 causes of group I ruled out	+1
		• 5 or 4 causes of group I ruled out	0
		• Less than 4 causes of group I ruled out	−2
		• Non drug cause highly probable	−3
6. PREVIOUS INFORMATION ON HEPATOTOXICITY OF THE DRUG			
Reaction labelled in the product characteristics			+2
Reaction published but unlabelled			+1
Reaction unknown			0
7. RESPONSE TO READMINISTRATION			
Positive	Doubling of ALT with the drug alone	Doubling of AP (or TB) with the drug alone	+3
Compatible	Doubling of ALT with the drugs already given at the time of the 1st reaction	Doubling of AP (or TB) with the drugs already given at the time of the 1st reaction	+1
Negative	Increase of ALT but less than N in the same conditions as for the first administration	Increase of AP (or TB) but less than N in the same conditions as for the first administration	−2
Not done or not interpretable	Other situations	Other situations	0
		TOTAL (add the circled figures)	

Reproduced with the permission of Roussel Uclaf

Application of RUCAM to acute liver injuries

The criteria for drug-induced liver injuries (Figure 2) have the following characteristics:

- the *time to onset* is never considered as highly suggestive or inconclusive. The causal relationship can be assessed as "unrelated" when the reaction occurred before the start of treatment or more than 15 days after stopping the treatment in case of hepatocellular injury, and more than 30 days in case of cholestatic or mixed type. When it is not possible to ascertain that the reaction occurred after the treatment was initiated or less than 15 or 30 days, depending on the type, after the discontinuation of the drug, the case report can be assessed as "insufficiently documented."
- the *course of the reaction* is inconclusive when the drug is continued, since liver test abnormalities may return to normal despite the continuation of the offending drug.
- the *risk factors* are:

  - age of patient over 55 years; whatever the type of liver damage, age seems to be a risk factor even after *adjustment for multiple drug consumption* which is associated with older patients;
  - alcohol consumption for hepatocellular type and alcohol consumption and/or pregnancy for cholestatic or mixed type.

- to date, there is no consensus for a laboratory test sensitive or specific enough to confirm the drug-related nature of a liver injury.
- The *"non drug-related causes"* to be sought have been divided into two groups. The first group consists of six causes with corresponding arguments:

  - IgM anti-HAV antibody indicates recent infection with hepatitis A virus (HAV);
  - IgM anti-HBc antibody indicates recent infection with hepatitis B virus (HBV);
  - non-A, non-B hepatitis: anti-hepatitis C virus (HCV) antibody (which may be present only after 1 or 2 months—sometimes 4 months—following the acute phase of liver injury), and circumstantial arguments including administration of blood or blood products 1–6 months previously, or recent travel to areas where hepatitis is endemic;
  - alcohol-induced injury is suggested when the ratio AST/ALT $\geqslant 2$;
  - ultrasonography of the liver and biliary tract looking for cholelithiasis or biliary tract abnormalities;
  - an episode of recent acute hypotension, leading to ischemic liver necrosis.

However, it is recognized that the role of HAV virus is unlikely in elderly patients, that ultrasonography of the liver is a mandatory diagnostic procedure in patients with cholestatic or mixed liver injury and that acute recent hypotension should mainly be investigated in specific circumstances such as arrhythmias, congestive heart failure and coronary insufficiency.

The search for the second group of causes is optional, depending on the clinical and/or biological context: natural history of the underlying disease and recent infection with cytomegalovirus (CMV), Epstein–Barr Virus (EBV) or herpes virus.

The search for the second group of causes is optional, depending on the clinical and/or biological context: natural history of the underlying disease and recent infection with cytomegalovirus (CMV), Epstein–Barr Virus (EBV) or herpes virus.

Comments

This novel method for drug causality assessment provides a standardized scoring system in which limits and contents of most of the criteria have been established by a consensus of experts.

The lack of reproducibility of most existing methods, i.e. disagreements between assessors, may be explained by the fact that the limits of criteria such as the timing of events, or the list of major alternative etiologies to be sought, are left up to each assessor's judgment (18). This judgment depends on each assessor's state of information when it should actually depend on information available in data banks, particularly epidemiological ones, but which unfortunately are often lacking.

Using RUCAM and the results of the Consensus Meetings, the time intervals have been strictly defined. The part left to the interpretation of the assessor is reduced, improving reproducibility. So does the standardization of the search for non drug-related causes, of the assessment of rechallenge and of the listing of risk factors.

References

Bénichou C, Danan G, Flahault A. Causality assessment of adverse reactions to drugs II. An original model for validation of drug causality assessment methods: case reports with positive rechallenge. Journal of Clinical Epidemiology 1993; 46: 1331–1336.

Danan G, Bénichou C. Causality assessment of adverse reactions to drugs I. A novel method based on the conclusions of international consensus meetings: application to drug-induced liver injuries. Journal of Clinical Epidemiology 1993; 46: 1323–1330.

APPENDIX
Specific Forms

	1. Identification n°/ Country	2. DRUG	3. Date of this report:
ADVERSE REACTION LIVER INJURY	4. CLINICAL TRIAL ☐ no ☐ yes Protocol n°: Centre n°: Patient:		5. REPORTER Name: Address: Tel.:

I. THE PATIENT

6. INITIALS (first, last):	7. SEX:	8. AGE	9. WEIGHT:
10. OCCUPATION:	11. COUNTRY OF ORIGIN:		12. OTHER:

13. PREVIOUS RELEVANT HISTORY AND CONCURRENT DISORDERS:

	no	yes	Specify		no	yes	Specify		no	yes
Current pregnancy	☐	☐		Cancer	☐	☐		Occupational toxic agent	☐	☐
Hepato-biliary	☐	☐		Surgical operation (dental)	☐	☐		Specify:		
Allergic disease	☐	☐		Date:				Travels: Africa, Asia	☐	☐
Allergy to drug	☐	☐		Transfusion of blood or derivatives	☐	☐				
Auto-Immune	☐	☐		Date:				Intravenous drug abuse	☐	☐
Heart/vascular diseases	☐	☐		Alcohol, consumption	☐	☐		Other:		
Respiratory	☐	☐		Acupuncture	☐	☐	date:			

II. THE ADVERSE REACTION   III. SUSPECTED DRUG

14. DATE OF ONSET	15. NATURE OF FIRST SYMPTOMS	21. Name

16. DESCRIPTION

	no	yes	Date		no	yes	Date		no	yes	Date
Asthenia	☐	☐		Abdominal pain	☐	☐		Hepatomegaly	☐	☐	
Fever	☐	☐		Vomiting	☐	☐		Splenomegaly	☐	☐	
Pruritis	☐	☐		Skin eruption	☐	☐		Lymph nodes	☐	☐	
Jaundice	☐	☐		type:				Ascites	☐	☐	
Joint pain	☐	☐						Asterixis	☐	☐	
				Purpura	☐	☐		Coma	☐	☐	

22. Indication

23. Daily dose

24. Route

17. LABORATORY DATA–Before/During/After treatment
(if necessary, continue overleaf)

DATES			
SGOT/SGPT (N< /)			
Alkaline Ph. (N<)			
GGT (N<)			
CPK (N<)			
Bilirubin			
Conjugated bilirubin			
γglobulins (g/l)			
P.T. (%)			
Factor V (%)			
Hemoglobin (g/dl)			
Leukocytes			
PMN			
Eosinos			
Creatininemia (units)			
Urea			

18. ULTRASONOGRAPHY
☐ no   ☐ yes   Date:

☐ normal

☐ abnormal *(brief results)*

19. LIVER BIOPSY
☐ no   ☐ yes   Date:

Results
(attach report)

25. Date beginning

26. Date end

27. Duration

28. ADMINISTRATION OF THE DRUG AFTER THE BEGINNING OF THE REACTION
☐ Stopped
☐ Continued (same dose)
☐ Reduced (dose):
☐ Other:

29. IMMEDIATE RESULT
☐ Improvement   ☐ No change
☐ Aggregation   ☐ Uninterpretable

Dates	Not tested	Absent	Present	Titre
HBs Ag	☐	☐	☐	
Anti-Hbs Ab	☐	☐	☐	
Anti-HBc Ab	☐	☐	☐	
Anti-Hbc/IgM Ab	☐	☐	☐	
Anti-HAV/IgM Ab	☐	☐	☐	
Anti-HCV Ab	☐	☐	☐	
Anti-CMV IgM Ab	☐	☐	☐	
Anti-EBV Ab	☐	☐	☐	
Anti nuclear Ab	☐	☐	☐	
Antinative DNA Ab	☐	☐	☐	
Anti-smooth muscle Ab	☐	☐	☐	
Antimitochondria Ab	☐	☐	☐	

20. OUTCOME *(tick more than one box if necessary)*
☐ no hospitalization   ☐ complete recovery
☐ Hospitalization necessary   ☐ Recovery with
address: sequelae

☐ Prolonged hospitalization

☐ Death   date:
Cause:

Relationship between the reaction and the death
☐ Not assessable   ☐ Unlikely   ☐ likely

30. READMINISTRATION OF THE DRUG
☐ no
☐ yes   dose: date:
and, if yes:

31. RECURRENCE OF THE REACTION
☐ no ☐ yes, date
☐ Uninterpretable

32. PREVIOUS THERAPY WITH THE SAME DRUG
☐ no ☐ yes, date
Safety issues:

IV. CONCOMITANT THERAPY *(continue overleaf if necessary)*

33. DRUGS	Route	Daily dose	Duration	Dates of administration		Indications
				Beginning	End	

34. CAUSAL RELATIONSHIP: ☐ Not assessable   ☐ Unrelated   ☐ Unlikely   ☐ Possible   ☐ Probable   ☐ Highly probable
(Reporter's assessment)

35. Has this case been reported to a Regulatory Agency?   ☐ No   ☐ Yes   To whom?   Date:

.... Cont'd→

	1. Identification N°/ Country	2. DRUG	3. DATE OF THIS REPORT:
ADVERSE REACTION HEMOLYSIS	4. CLINICAL TRIAL Protocol n°: Centre n°:	☐ no ☐ yes Patient:	5. REPORTER Name: Address: Tel.:

I. THE PATIENT

6. INITIALS (first, last):   7. SEX: 8. AGE   9. WEIGHT:

10. OCCUPATION   11. COUNTRY OF ORIGIN: 12. OTHER:

13. PREVIOUS RELEVANT HISTORY:

	No	Yes	Specify (HBs, G6PD)			No	Yes	Specify
HEREDITARY HEMOLYSIS:	☐	☐		Allergic disease		☐	☐	
Patient ☐				Allergy to drug		☐	☐	
Family ☐				Other Specify				

II. THE ADVERSE REACTION *(continue overleaf if necessary)*   III. SUSPECTED DRUG

14. DATE OF ONSET: Precise exact time: | 15. NATURE OF FIRST SIGNS:

21. Name

16. DESCRIPTION

	No	Yes		No	Yes	Other (specify)
Lumbar pain	☐	☐	Splenomegaly	☐	☐	
Abdominal pain	☐	☐	Fever	☐	☐	
Bone pain	☐	☐	Shock/collapsus	☐	☐	
Headache	☐	☐	Jaundice	☐	☐	
			Black/red urine	☐	☐	
			Anuria	☐	☐	

22. Indication

23. Daily dose

24. Route

25. Date beginning

26. Date end

27. Duration

17. LABORATORY DATA: Before/during/after treatment
DATES

Hemoglobin
MCV
Reticulocytes
Erythrocyte abnormalities
Leucocytes
Platelets
Bilirubin (units)
Haptoglobin
Hemoglobinemia
SGOT/SGPT (N= /)
LDH (N=)
BUN
Creatininemia
PT (patient/control)
APTT (patient/control)

28. ADMINISTRATION OF THE DRUG AFTER THE BEGINNING OF THE REACTION
☐ Stopped
☐ Continued (same dose)
☐ Reduced dose:
☐ Other:

29. IMMEDIATE RESULT
☐ Improvement   ☐ No change
☐ Aggravation   ☐ Uninterpretable

30. READMINISTRATION OF THE DRUG
☐ No
☐ Yes, and if yes:

18. OTHER LABORATORY DATA

	Not done	Negative	Positive	Date
Coombs' test	☐	☐	☐	
Indirect Coombs' test	☐	☐	☐	
Anti-drug antibody	☐	☐	☐	
Cold agglutinin	☐	☐	☐	
	Titre:			
Serum freezing	☐ no	☐ yes, date:		

IF POSITIVE COOMBS TEST
TYPE: ☐ IgC   ☐ C ☐ IgC+C
SPECIFICITY: ☐ Rh (specify Rh antigen: Rh...)
☐ II   ☐ Other, specify
☐ Undetermined
    ☐ Not tested
Other laboratory data

31. RECURRENCE OF THE REACTION
☐ No   ☐ Yes
☐ Uninterpretable

32. PREVIOUS THERAPY WITH THE SAME DRUG
☐ No   ☐ Yes

Safety issues:

19. TREATMENT OF THE HEMOLYSIS AND/OR ITS COMPLICATIONS *(specify doses and duration)*
☐ Steroids
☐ Plasma exchanges
☐ Hemodialysis
☐ RBC transfusions, dates:
☐ Other, specify

20. OUTCOME *(Tick more than one if necessary)*
☐ No hospitalization
☐ Hospitalization necessary
   Address
☐ Prolonged hospitalization
☐ Complete recovery
☐ Recovery with sequelae (specify):

Death   date:
    Cause
Relationship between the reaction and the death
☐ Not assessable   ☐ Unlikely
☐ Likely

IV. CONCOMITANT THERAPY *(continue overleaf if necessary)*

33. DRUGS	Route	Daily dose	Duration	Dates of administration		Indications
				Beginning	End	

34. CAUSAL RELATIONSHIP: ☐ Not assessable   ☐ Unrelated   ☐ Unlikely   ☐ Possible   ☐ Probable   ☐ Highly probable
(Reporter's assessment)

35. Has this case been reported to a Regulatory Agency?   ☐ No   ☐ Yes   To whom?   Date:

Reproduced with the permission of Roussel Uclaf.   .... Cont'd→

ADVERSE REACTION KIDNEY DISORDERS	1. Identification N°/ Country	2. DRUG	3. DATE OF THIS REPORT:
			5. REPORTER Name:
	4. CLINICAL TRIAL Protocol n°: ☐ no ☐ yes		Address:
	Centre n°: Patient:		Tel.:

I. THE PATIENT

6. INITIALS (first, last):   7. SEX: 8. AGE   9. WEIGHT:
10. OCCUPATION: 11. COUNTRY OF ORIGIN: 12. OTHER:

13. PREVIOUS RELEVANT HISTORY: No   Yes   Specify

	No	Yes	Specify		No	Yes	Specify
				Preexisting nephropathy	☐	☐	
Current pregnancy	☐	☐		Urological history	☐	☐	
Hypertension	☐	☐		Allergy to drugs	☐	☐	
Cardiac failure	☐	☐		Diabetes	☐	☐	
Hepatocellular failure	☐	☐		Other			

II. THE ADVERSE REACTION *(continue overleaf if necessary)*

III. SUSPECTED DRUG

14. DATE OF ONSET: 15. NATURE OF FIRST SIGNS:

16. DESCRIPTION:

	No	Yes	Date		No	Yes	Date		No	Yes	Date
Oliguria	☐	☐		Hypertension	☐	☐		Eruption	☐	☐	
Anuria	☐	☐		Dehydration	☐	☐		Joint pain	☐	☐	
Lumbar pain	☐	☐		Collapse/shock	☐	☐		Jaundice	☐	☐	
Macro. hematuria	☐	☐		Fever	☐	☐		Purpura	☐	☐	
Edema	☐	☐						Other			

17. LABORATORY DATA: Before/during/after treatment

	DATES							
B L O O D	Creatinin							
	BUN							
	Total protein							
	Albumin							
	Na/K							
	Bicarbonate							
	Ca/P							
	Hemoglobin							
	Leukocytes							
	Eosinos							
	Platelets							
	Alk Phosph.*							
	SGOT/SGPT*							
	Creatine Kinase*							
	BSR							
U R I N E	Daily output							
	Creatinine/l							
	Proteinuria/24 h							
	Hematuria							
	Leukocytes							
	Na/K							
	Cristalluria							

*Give the normal values

III. SUSPECTED DRUG (right column)

21. Name

22. Indication

23. Daily dose

24. Route

25. Date beginning

26. Date end

27. Duration

28. ADMINISTRATION OF THE DRUG AFTER THE BEGINNING OF THE REACTION
☐ Stopped
☐ Continued (same dose)
☐ Reduced dose:
☐ Other:

29. IMMEDIATE RESULT
☐ Improvement   ☐ No change
☐ Aggravation   ☐ Uninterpretable

30. READMINISTRATION OF THE DRUG
☐ No
☐ Yes, and if yes:

31. RECURRENCE OF THE REACTION
☐ No   ☐ Yes
☐ Uninterpretable

32. PREVIOUS THERAPY WITH THE SAME DRUG
☐ No   ☐ Yes
Safety issues:

18. OTHER LABORATORY DATA

	(*) ND	N	A	Specify
Urine culture	☐	☐	☐	
IVP	☐	☐	☐	
Renal sonography	☐	☐	☐	
Eosinophiluria	☐	☐	☐	

☐ RENAL BIOPSY   date
Result (attach histology report)
*(NC): Not Done (N): Normal · (A): Abnormal

☐ IMMUNOLOGICAL TESTS (Specify):
Results *(continue overleaf if necessary)*

19. TREATMENT OF RENAL DISORDERS   ☐ Steroids   ☐ Transient dialysis   ☐ Chronic dialysis
☐ Other *(specify)*

20. OUTCOME *(tick more than one box if necessary)*   ☐ Death   date:
☐ No hospitalization   ☐ Complete recovery   Cause:
☐ Hospitalization necessary   ☐ Recovery with sequelae   Relationship between the reaction
address   specify: and the death
☐ Prolonged hospitalization   ☐ Not assessable   ☐ Unlikely   ☐ Likely

IV. CONCOMITANT THERAPY *(continue overleaf if necessary)*

33. DRUGS	Route	Daily dose	Duration	Dates of administration		Indications
				Beginning	End	

34. CAUSAL RELATIONSHIP: ☐ Not assessable   ☐ Unrelated   ☐ Unlikely   ☐ Possible   ☐ Probable   ☐ Highly probable
(Reporter's assessment)

35. Has this case been reported to a Regulatory Agency?   ☐ No   ☐ Yes   To whom?   Date:

Reproduced with the permission of Roussel Uclaf.   . . . . Cont'd→

ADVERSE REACTION
THROMBOCYTOPENIA

1. Identification N°/ Country	2. DRUG

3. DATE OF THIS REPORT:

5. REPORTER
Name:

4. CLINICAL TRIAL   ☐ no   ☐ yes
Protocol n°:
Centre n°:   Patient:

Address:

Tel.:

I. THE PATIENT

6. INITIALS (first, last):   7. SEX: 8. AGE   9. WEIGHT:
10. OCCUPATION: 11. COUNTRY OF ORIGIN: 12. OTHER:

13. PREVIOUS RELEVANT HISTORY:

	No	Yes	Specify
Hematological-Oncological	☐	☐	
Allergic reactions	☐	☐	
Drug intolerance	☐	☐	
Alcohol	☐	☐	

Other:

II. THE ADVERSE REACTION *(continue overleaf if necessary)*

III. SUSPECTED DRUG

14. DATE OF ONSET: 15. NATURE OF FIRST SIGNS:

21. Name

16. DESCRIPTION:

	No	Yes		No	Yes		No	Yes	Date
			Genital bleeding	☐	☐	Fever	☐	☐	
Purpura	☐	☐	Cerebro-meningeal bleeding	☐	☐	Jaundice	☐	☐	
Epistaxis	☐	☐				Infection	☐	☐	
Gingivorrhagia	☐	☐	Retinal bleeding	☐	☐	Other:	☐	☐	
GI bleeding	☐	☐	Other-bleeding Specify			Specify			

22. Indication

23. Daily dose

24. Route

17. LABORATORY DATA: Before/during/after treatment
DATES

Platelets					
Hemoglobin					
Reticulocytes					
Leukocytes					
PMN (%)					
BLEEDING TIME*					
APTT (Pt/control)					
PT (%)					
SGOT/SGPT**					

* Method and normal range
**Normal range (NE   /   )

25. Date beginning

26. Date end

27. Duration

28. ADMINISTRATION OF THE DRUG AFTER THE BEGINNING OF THE REACTION
☐ Stopped
☐ Continued (same dose)
☐ Reduced dose:
☐ Other:

29. IMMEDIATE RESULT
☐ Improvement ☐ No change
☐ Aggravation ☐ Uninterpretable

18. OTHER LABORATORY DATA
☐ Bone marrow aspiration   Date:
    Cellularity
    Megakaryocytes
    ☐ Increased ☐ Normal ☐ Decreased
☐ Platelet associated Immunoglob. Date
    Methods and normal
    Results:

	(*) N.D.	Neg.	Pos.	
Blood culture	☐	☐	☐	Germ:
R.B.C. Coomb's test	☐	☐	☐	Type:
Anti-nuclear antibodies	☐	☐	☐	Type:
HIV Serology	☐	☐	☐	Method:
Other serologies	☐	☐	☐	Virus:
				Titre:

SERUM FREEZING   ☐ No ☐ Yes, date
OTHERS:
(*) N.D.=Not done Neg.=negative Pos.=positive

30. READMINISTRATION OF THE DRUG
☐ No
☐ Yes, and if yes:

31. RECURRENCE OF THE REACTION
☐ No   ☐ Yes
☐ Uninterpretable

32. PREVIOUS THERAPY WITH THE SAME DRUG
☐ No   ☐ Yes
Safety issues:

19. TREATMENT OF THE THROMBOCYTOPENIA AND/OR ITS COMPLICATIONS *(specify doses and duration)*

☐ Steroids   ☐ Immunoglobulins
☐ RBC transfusion, dates   ☐ Other (specify)
☐ Platelet transfusion
. Dates
. Types

20. OUTCOME *(Tick more than one box if necessary)*
☐ No hospitalization
☐ Hospitalization necessary
    Address:

☐ Prolonged hospitalization
☐ Complete recovery
☐ Recovery with sequelae (specify):

☐ Death   date:
Cause:
Relationship between the reaction and the death
☐ Not assessable ☐ Unlikely
☐ Likely

IV. CONCOMITANT THERAPY *(continue overleaf if necessary)*

33. DRUGS	Route	Daily dose	Duration	Dates of administration		Indications
				Beginning	End	

34. CAUSAL RELATIONSHIP: ☐ Not assessable   ☐ Unrelated   ☐ Unlikely   ☐ Possible   ☐ Probable   ☐ Highly probable
(Reporter's assessment)

35. Has this case been reported to a Regulatory Agency?   ☐ No   ☐ Yes   To whom?   Date:

Reproduced with the permission of Roussel Uclaf.   . . . . Cont'd→

ADVERSE REACTION INTERNATIONAL REPORT FORM

1. Identification no/Country	2. DRUG	3. DATE OF THIS REPORT:

4. CLINICAL TRIAL	☐ No	☐ Yes	5. REPORTER NAME:
Protocol no:			Address:
Centre no:		Patient no:	Tel.:

I. THE PATIENT

6. INITIALS (first, last):	7. SEX:	8. AGE:	9. WEIGHT:
10. OCCUPATION:	11. COUNTRY OF ORIGIN:		

12. PREVIOUS RELEVANT HISTORY

13. PREVIOUS INTOLERANCE TO DRUGS ☐ No ☐ Yes to what drug:

II. THE ADVERSE REACTION *(continue overleaf if necessary)*

14. DATE REACTION OCCURRED:

15. time-interval after the last intake of the drug:

16. DESCRIPTION, SEARCH FOR NON DRUG CAUSES, AND RELEVANT LABORATORY OR OTHER EXAMINATIONS DATA (WITH DATES):

17. TREATMENT OF THE REACTION

18. EVOLUTION *(Tick more than one box if necessary)*

☐ No hospitalization

☐ Hospitalization necessary   ☐ Complete recovery
Address:
                                ☐ Recovery with sequelae
☐ Prolonged hospitalization

☐ Death   date:
Cause:
Relationship between the reaction
and the death
☐ Not assessable   ☐ Unlikely
☐ likely

III. SUSPECTED DRUG

19. Name

20. Indication

21. Daily dose

22. Route

23. Date beginning

24. Date end

25. Duration

26. ADMINISTRATION OF THIS DRUG AFTER THE BEGINNING OF THE REACTION
☐ Stopped
☐ Continued (same dose)
☐ Reduced dose:
☐ Other:

27. IMMEDIATE RESULT
☐ Improvement ☐ No change
☐ Aggravation ☐ Uninterpretable

28. READMINISTRATION OF THE DRUG
☐ No
☐ Yes, and if yes
dose:
date:

29. RECURRENCE OF THE REACTION
☐ No ☐ Yes
☐ Uninterpretable

30. PREVIOUS THERAPY WITH THE SAME DRUG
☐ No ☐ Yes, date:
Safety issues:

IV. CONCOMITANT THERAPY *(continue overleaf if necessary)*

31. DRUGS	Route	Daily dose	Duration	Dates of administration		Indications
				Beginning	End	

32. CAUSAL RELATIONSHIP *(Reporter's assessment):*   ☐ Not assessable ☐ Unrelated ☐ Unlikely ☐ Possible ☐ Probable ☐ Highly probable

33. Has this case been reported to a Regulatory Agency? ☐ No ☐ Yes To whom?: Date:

Reproduced with the permission of Roussel Uclaf

ADVERSE REACTION
NEUTROPENIA

1. Identification no/Country	2. DRUG	3. DATE OF THIS REPORT:

4. CLINICAL TRIAL ☐ No ☐ Yes	5. REPORTER
Protocol no:	NAME:
	Address:
Centre no: Patient no:	Tel.:

I. THE PATIENT

6. INITIALS (first, last):	7. SEX:	8. AGE	9. WEIGHT:
10. OCCUPATION:	11. COUNTRY OF ORIGIN:		12. OTHER:

13. PREVIOUS RELEVANT HISTORY:

	No	Yes	Specify	Other:
Haematological—Oncological	☐	☐		
Allergic reactions	☐	☐		
Drug allergy	☐	☐		

II. THE ADVERSE REACTION *(continue overleaf if necessary)*

III. SUSPECTED DRUG

14. DATE OF ONSET:	15. NATURE OF FIRST SIGNS:

16. DESCRIPTION:

	No	Yes		No	Yes	BLOOD CULTURES
Fever	☐	☐	Oropharyngeal ulcerations	☐	☐	☐ Not done ☐ Negative
Collapsus/shock	☐	☐	Perineal ulcerations	☐	☐	☐ Positive
Infection	☐	☐	Other symptoms:			germs:
Localization						Dates:

17. LABORATORY DATA: before/during/after treatment
DATES

Leukocytes					
PMN (%)					
Eosinos (%)					
Lymphocytes (%)					
Monocytes (%)					
Platelets					
Hemoglobin (units)					
Reticulocytes					
Total bilirubin					
SGOT/SGPT (N= /)					

BONE MARROW ASPIRATION(S), DATES
Cellularity
% Myeloid cells
% Other cells *(specify)*

18. OTHER LABORATORY DATA

	Negative	Positive	Not done
Antineutrophil antibodies	☐	☐	☐

Serum freezing ☐ No   ☐ Yes   Date:

Bone marrow
Precursor cell culture   ☐ No   ☐ Yes
Date
If yes, attach the results

BONE MARROW BIOPSY   ☐ No   ☐ Yes
Results *(attach pathological report)*

19. TREATMENT OF THE NEUTROPENIA AND/OR ITS
COMPLICATIONS *(specify doses and duration)*

☐ Growth factors (G-CSF, GM-CSF)

☐ Steroids

☐ Antibiotics

☐ Other, specify:

20. OUTCOME *(tick more than one box if necessary)*
☐ No hospitalization
☐ Hospitalization necessary
   Address:
☐ Prolonged hospitalization
☐ Complete recovery
☐ Recovery with sequelae *(specify)*:

III. SUSPECTED DRUG

21. Name

22. Indication

23. Daily dose

24. Route

25. Date beginning

26. Date end

27. Duration

28. ADMINISTRATION OF THIS DRUG AFTER
THE BEGINNING OF THE REACTION
☐ Stopped
☐ Continued (same dose)
☐ Reduced dose:
☐ Other:

29. IMMEDIATE RESULT
☐ Improvement ☐ No change
☐ Aggravation ☐ Uninterpretable

30. READMINISTRATION OF THE DRUG
☐ No
☐ Yes, and if yes
31. RECURRENCE OF THE REACTION
☐ No ☐ Yes, date
☐ Uninterpretable:

32. PREVIOUS THERAPY WITH THE
SAME DRUG
☐ No ☐ Yes, date:
Safety issues:

☐ Death   date:
Cause:
Relationship between the reaction
and the death
☐ Not assessable   ☐ Unlikely
☐ likely

IV. CONCOMITANT THERAPY *(continue overleaf if necessary)*

33. DRUGS	Route	Daily dose	Duration	Dates of administration		Indications
				Beginning	End	

34. CAUSAL RELATIONSHIP
(Reporter's assessment):
☐ Not assessable   ☐ Unrelated   ☐ Unlikely   ☐ Possible   ☐ Probable   ☐ Highly probable

33. Has this case been reported to a Regulatory Agency?   ☐ No   ☐ Yes   To whom?:   Date:

Reproduced with the permission of Roussel Uclaf

ADVERSE REACTION SKIN DISORDERS

1. Identification no/Country	2. DRUG	3. DATE OF THIS REPORT:

4. CLINICAL TRIAL   ☐ No ☐ Yes
Protocol no:
Centre no: Patient no:

5. REPORTER
NAME:
Address:
Tel.:
Dermatologist ☐ Yes ☐ No

I. THE PATIENT

6. INITIALS (first, last):   7. SEX: 8. AGE   9. WEIGHT:

10. OCCUPATION: 11. COUNTRY OF ORIGIN: 12. OTHER:

13. PREVIOUS RELEVANT HISTORY AND CONCURRENT DISORDERS:
           No   Yes   Specify:
Skin diseases   ☐   ☐
Other diseases   ☐   ☐

Allergic reactions ☐   Specify:
to what drug?

Asthma ☐   Allergic rhinitis ☐   Atopic dermatitis ☐

II. THE ADVERSE REACTION (continue overleaf if necessary)

14. DATE OF ONSET: 15. NATURE OF FIRST SIGNS:

16. TYPE OF SKIN DISORDER
☐ Macular or maculopapular rash
☐ Scarlatiniform rash
☐ Exfoliative dermatitis
☐ Bullous or vesiculous eruption
Specify: ☐ Fixed drug eruption
    ☐ Erythema multiforme (target lesions)
    ☐ Stevens-Johnson syndrome
    ☐ Toxic Epidermal Necrolysis (TEN)
    ☐ Other:
☐ Purpura (platelet count needed)
    ☐ palpable purpura ☐ necrotic purpura
    ☐ visceral involvement:
       ☐ Kidney ☐ GI tract ☐ Nerves
       ☐ Others:

☐ Pruritus alone
☐ Contact dermatitis or eczematiform eruption
☐ Urticaria
☐ Cutaneous angioedema
☐ Mucosal angioedema

associated signs: ☐ Dyspnea
              ☐ Tachycardia
              ☐ Hypotension
              ☐ Anaphylactic shock

☐ Other skin disorders, (specify):

Were photographs taken? ☐ No Yes   Are duplicata available? ☐ No ☐ Yes

17. DISTRIBUTION OF LESIONS   ☐ localized   ☐ disseminated
Number of lesions ☐ < 10 ☐ 10 to 30 ☐ > 30   main location:
☐ Mucosal lesions, specify:
☐ Nail/hair lesions, specify:

18. ASSOCIATED SYMPTOMS
☐ Pruritus   ☐ Fever
☐ Burning or pain   ☐ Arthralgia/myalgia
☐ Oozing   ☐ Nodes enlargement
☐ Edema
☐ Infection   ☐ Other, specify:

Evidence for viral infection: No   Yes   Not done
EBV   ☐   ☐   ☐
Hepatitis B virus   ☐   ☐   ☐
CMV   ☐   ☐   ☐
Herpes   ☐   ☐   ☐
HIV   ☐   ☐   ☐
Other:

19. IS PHOTOSENSITIVITY SUSPECTED?   ☐ No ☐ Yes
.Localization of lesion: ☐ Face ☐ Neck ☐ Hands/forearms
                   ☐ Legs/feet ☐ Other specify:
.Intensity of solar exposition: ☐ High ☐ Mild ☐ Low

20. LABORATORY DATA
.Leucocytes:
.PMNs: %
.Eosinophils: &
.Platelets:
.ESR:
.ALT/AST: (N = /)
.Alk.Ph.:   (N = /)

SKIN BIOPSY: ☐ No ☐ Yes
Result (attach report)

IMMUNOFLUORESCENT STAINING:
            ☐ No ☐ Yes
Result (attach report)

22. OUTCOME
(tick more than one box if necessary)
☐ No hospitalization
☐ Hospitalization necessary
   address:
☐ Prolonged hospitalization
☐ Complete recovery
☐ Recovery with sequelae (specify):

21. TREATMENT OF REACTION ☐ No ☐ Yes (continue overleaf)

III. SUSPECTED DRUG

23. Name

24. Indication

25. Daily dose

26. Route

27. Date beginning

28. Date end

29. Duration

30. ADMINISTRATION OF THIS DRUG AFTER THE BEGINNING OF THE REACTION
☐ Stopped
☐ Continued (same dose)
☐ Reduced dose:
☐ Other:

31. IMMEDIATE RESULT
☐ Improvement ☐ No change
☐ Aggravation ☐ Uninterpretable

32. READMINISTRATION OF THE DRUG
☐ No   ☐ Yes
Dose: Date:
and if yes:

33. RECURRENCE OF THE REACTION
☐ No ☐ Yes,
☐ Uninterpretable:

34. PREVIOUS THERAPY WITH THE SAME DRUG
☐ No ☐ Yes, date:
Safety issues:

☐ Death   date:
   Cause:
Relationship between the reaction and the death
☐ Not assessable
☐ Unlikely
☐ Likely

IV. CONCOMITANT THERAPY (continue overleaf if necessary)

35. DRUGS	Route	Daily dose	Duration	Dates of administration		Indications
				Beginning	End	

36. CAUSAL RELATIONSHIP   ☐ Not assessable ☐ Unrelated ☐ Unlikely ☐ Possible ☐ Probable ☐ Highly probable
(Reporter's assessment):

37. Has this case been reported to a Regulatory Agency?   ☐ No   ☐ Yes   To whom?:   Date:

Index

Compiled by Geoffrey C. Jones